THE DEMENTIA CAREGIVER'S HANDBOOK

THE SEVEN STAGES AND HOW TO NAVIGATE
FINANCIAL STRUGGLES, OVERCOME ISOLATION, AND
UNDERSTAND THE CHANGES IN YOUR LOVED ONE
WITHOUT FEELING GUILT OR REMORSE

ROSALIND BAKER-WARREN

CONTENTS

INTRODUCTION

Have you ever walked into a room, stopped for a second, and then remembered what you went there for? Just imagine that happening every day, in all situations, and basically all the time; then, you will have some idea of what is going on with your loved one who has dementia.

Your brain has nerves that "talk" to each other via links. When the link is broken, lapses occur. In a modern world context, we can compare it to your internet connection. If there is a break in the cable, your internet signal will be lost because it can't jump over a lost link. As more links in the brain start to malfunction, dementia grows.

And now let's talk about you, the caregiver. Whether you are the only caregiver or if you get some support from family members or outside help, the bulk of the care comes from you. Your burnout is a very real possibility, and because maybe you are holding down a job and you have other family responsibilities, it is likely that you won't even realize you are burning out until it is almost too late.

As a caregiver to someone with dementia, it is essential that you understand the ramifications so that you can take care of yourself on this unsettling journey. If you totally fall to pieces under the stress, you will be pretty useless to your loved one.

I am writing this book to help you understand the condition you are nursing. I will go through the seven stages, explaining carefully what you can expect. Forewarned is forearmed (*King James Bible*, 2017/1769, I Corinthians 10).

During my discussions with you, I will give you helpful advice because I know what you are going through. I have been there, and it can sometimes be a rocky road, but with knowledge comes understanding. The understanding will give you the tools you need to travel this road with your loved one.

WHO IS ROSALIND BAKER-WARREN?

I gleaned a lot while Mom and I were caring for my dad during the dementia that eventually took him away from us. No one ever tells you what dementia does to the body, as well as the mind. We tried to keep him at home with us for as long as we could. The balancing act 24/7 is exhausting physically, mentally, emotionally, and spiritually. It is a lonely road, even if you have someone else to share the burden. I had to keep an eye on my mother as well to make sure that she didn't crumble under the stress.

It is sometimes difficult to accept and run with the changes that come with dementia without losing your cool. I had to continually remind myself that it was the disease, not my father, when he couldn't remember things or participate in conversations around him.

We watched as friends and some family members decided to stay away rather than support us while we fended off stupid questions and beliefs. I can't remember how many times I had to say things like "No, it is not contagious," "No, God is not going to miraculously heal him," and "Yes, I sometimes worry it is hereditary." I came away with the unsettling thought, *Will this be me in years to come?*

More stress and uncertainty came when we finally had to put him in a place where he would receive the care that he needed and we could no longer give. We also had to face the fact that this would be an expensive experience. Sticker shock doesn't begin to describe the cost of long-term care. And the emotional toll of navigating a seriously flawed elder care system is exhausting. I examined many options but every single one of them fell short of my expectations to a lesser or greater degree. So eventually, I took the one that seemed to come closest to my expectations.

The first time I told a friend about my dad's diagnosis, I watched him flinch before telling me he had been a caregiver for his own father for many years. He hesitated, then told me that for three years he was angry with his dad, three years he was angry with God, then for three years he was angry at himself. I've never heard a more accurate portrayal of what the caregiver goes through.

I had an overwhelming desire to share my turmoil and, in so doing, alleviate some of the stress that you, the reader, may be feeling. I also wanted to share my knowledge which is the product of sitting, sometimes well into the night, researching this disease that had been visited on my family. This book is the outcome of all these desires, heartache, and research.

ABOUT THE BOOK

As has already been described, I want to help you have as positive an experience as possible.

- Chapter 1 helps you understand dementia as well as the subtypes of dementia. The seven stages of dementia will be explained briefly. It is rather long and involved but gives you a good picture of what your loved one is going through.
- Chapter 2 discusses the first three stages of dementia, often called pre-dementia. These stages usually occur prior to being medically diagnosed. The symptoms could be confused with normal aging

symptoms. You may be developing concerns as to whether these are, in fact, aligned with dementia, or your loved one has already been diagnosed with dementia and you need to fill in gaps and give yourself "aha" moments as you recognize the symptoms in retrospect.

- Chapter 3 deals with the 4th stage of dementia. Your loved one has been diagnosed and you, the caregiver, can educate yourself as to what to expect and how to deal with it. You may like to hold off continuing reading until the fifth stage is reached or you may like to prepare yourself for the future. It is an entirely personal decision. If you put off reading further, do not wait too long before picking up again. You do not want to be in the full throes of the fifth stage without any preparation.

- Chapter 4 deals with the fifth stage of dementia. This is a hard one, as you may need to look for more substantial help with your loved one. There will be a noticeable decline in their memory and their ability to deal with everyday situations will decline. They will need increasing help to do tasks like dressing themselves.

- Chapter 5 helps you to understand the sixth stage of dementia. They will need a lot of help with normal living tasks. This can be exhausting for the caregiver and you may continually berate yourself for failing to help them. This is normal and you are not at fault.

- Chapter 6 helps you to understand that their time on earth is limited and you will need more input from health care providers. Your task will be to keep them comfortable until the end.
- Chapter 7 helps you deal with the aftermath of suddenly having no one to care for. Now is the time you need to grieve and pick up the pieces of your own life.
- Additional Resources can be found after the conclusion.

If there is one message I want every reader to take away from this book, it is this—wherever this journey takes you, *you are enough*!

AN OVERVIEW OF DEMENTIA

W henever we hear the word dementia, most of us will substitute "Alzheimer's" but there are many types of dementia, and Alzheimer's is just one of them. It is the most common type, the one we hear about most frequently, but there are a lot more different types of dementia. I will give you some insight into many types of dementia later in this chapter.

WHAT IS DEMENTIA?

- Dementia is a clump of diseases that affect the brain.
- All dementias are progressive diseases. Once it starts, it gets progressively worse.

- Dementia is not curable, although many types of dementia do have drugs that can mask or delay the symptoms.
- Scientists now believe that dementia starts at least 20 years before one experiences the first signs of it.

The brain is the most important organ in the body. It is the seat of control for all things that you do voluntarily or involuntarily.

THE BRAIN

The brain is a wonderful part of our body. It controls everything that we do, think, and experience. When a part of the brain gets damaged, whatever that part of the brain controls is likely to stop functioning or start malfunctioning.

The brain has billions of interconnected neurons that are continually sending messages to other parts of the brain and parts of the body. If, for example, the patient no longer understands how to brush his teeth, it is because the neurons in that part of the brain have broken connections. So the message is garbled, incomplete, or nonexistent. As the caregiver, you could take your loved one to the bathroom sink, put toothpaste on the brush, and give it to them and they would not know what to do with it. It is not their fault and no amount of begging, shouting, or crying will help them get that job completed.

In dementia, the damage to the neurons and their connections is permanent. We could almost say that the affected part of the brain has died. As the disease takes control, it is as if the neurons are acting like a set of standing dominoes. Tip the first domino over and set the destruction going. As the years, then the months count over, more and more neurons and their connections become unstable and eventually cease to work. The patient becomes increasingly incapable of thinking logically and doing simple everyday tasks. And the caregiver is taxed with the job of keeping them safe, thinking for them, and doing those simple everyday tasks for them.

FACTS FROM THE WORLD HEALTH ORGANISATION

- As of March this year, there are more than 55 million cases of dementia in the world. This number grows by about 10 million yearly.
- More than half of these cases are in middle to low-income areas.
- Dementia is the 7th most common cause of death.
- It adversely affects the wealth of countries as well as affected families.
- More women than men have dementia.
- More women than men become caregivers to dementia patients (World Health Organization, 2023).

SUBTYPES OF DEMENTIA

As mentioned earlier, dementia is a blanket term for many afflictions of the brain. Although when they hear the word dementia, most people only think of Alzheimer's. There are many other causes of dementia and each disease acts in a specific way. The patient's behavior is specific to the type of dementia, although there are a few similarities.

Alzheimer's Disease

Alois Alzheimer (1864–1915) was a German psychiatrist who discovered, diagnosed, and gave his name to this disease. Out of all the dementia diseases, this is the most common one. It affects the patient's memory and alters their behavior. Their ability to think tasks through is one of the most frustrating symptoms of this disease for their caregivers.

In America, it is estimated that 60–80% of all dementia patients are Alzheimer's patients who are being cared for by 11 million voluntary caregivers (Alzheimer's Association, 2023). It must be stressed that any dementia, and that includes Alzheimer's, is not a normal progression in old age.

As with all dementia, Alzheimer's degradation continues. It is not curable but there are medications that could slow down the progress of the disease. It is still a topic of research as scientists attempt to find ways to slow the disease down.

There are even studies that are examining the possibility of halting the disease.

Alzheimer's disease starts slowly many years before the first symptoms appear. The first signs are usually the inability to recall something that has just happened or that the patient has learned about recently. If a patient is told that their granddaughter got engaged, they will be delighted but will soon insist that nobody told them. A frequent chant will be, "Nobody ever tells me anything."

This memory loss causes them to ask the same question over and over again. At first, the family may feel that the patient just is not listening. But this is not the case; they have genuinely forgotten that they asked the question. It is essential that the caregiver does not lose patience. I know that it is very easy to say this, but the reality is hard, and the caregiver may find that they are continually biting their tongue to prevent their frustration from shining through.

The patient will rely more and more on the caregiver for tasks that were previously handled with ease. Financial items like paying the electricity bill will not be remembered and they could end up losing their utilities. While you, the caregiver, will have to take more responsibility for essential tasks, at this stage, try not to trample on their self-esteem and their vision of their independence.

Routines will become less familiar. Things they have done for years will become difficult. They may get lost traveling familiar routes. The role of the caregiver is difficult as they have to know when they need to interfere and take over. They must also take over in a friendly, coercive manner. Now is not the time to lose patience and shout, "Oh, let me do it." Rather have something like, "It is getting to that time of the month when we need to sort bills. Let me help you get them together" and then gently take over bit by bit. If you are worried about them getting lost when they drive, suggest that you give them a break from driving and you will take them wherever they want to go. You will probably meet with resistance the first few times but eventually, they will be quite pleased to hand the driving over to you. The progress of dementia will be discussed further later in the book. Right now, we are aiming to give you a picture of what you are facing and why.

As you observe your elderly loved one, you may be uncertain whether they are in the early stages of Alzheimer's or if it is just a symptom of aging. The only thing that will clearly establish the difference is a medical examination. This examination may include an MRI or a PET scan. You may also look at a DNA test to establish if that is in their DNA signature. If it runs in their family, then they stand a bigger chance of developing Alzheimer's but this is not a certainty. It is important to note that many people age normally and have no signs of dementia. They may forget people's names or other significant information only to remember it an hour or so later.

What Happens to the Brain?

An accumulation of the protein beta-amyloid around the neurons of the brain leads to the death of the neurons. The brain tissue in that area is damaged and this damage can be picked up during the scans.

A hallmark of Alzheimer's is that the neurons killed are in the area that houses memory. The spread of the disease is in a predictable pattern.

Types of Alzheimer's

There are two types of Alzheimer's:

- Early-onset Alzheimer's affects people below 60 years of age. It will often appear in a person's 30's. It is usually genetic and is not very common.
- Over 60's who are diagnosed with Alzheimer's are classified as having late-onset Alzheimer's.

Vascular Dementia

Vascular Dementia is often stroke-related, although it could originate in people with high blood pressure, diabetes, or high cholesterol. All three of these conditions could, in themselves, cause a stroke. I must, however, add that not all strokes lead to vascular dementia. It depends on where in the brain the stroke and damage occurred. And some cases of vascular dementia are not a result of a stroke (see the three other conditions mentioned in the first sentence of this paragraph). Smokers are also at risk of developing vascular dementia.

Whatever the causes, there is irreversible damage in the brain which will continue to get worse if the patient does not change their health habits. Exercise and a healthy diet can slow down the disease, as can controlling your blood pressure and cholesterol. If you are a smoker, now is the time to quit.

The brain is damaged during a stroke or a series of mini-strokes. A mini-stroke is actually called a transient ischemic attack (TIA) which lasts for a couple of minutes. One such stroke doesn't cause permanent damage, but if you have a series of them, there is a likelihood of damage occurring. If you have suffered a mini stroke, you are a likely candidate for a full stroke and it is time to do some drastic lifestyle changes.

The symptoms of vascular dementia usually occur rapidly after a stroke. They are similar to Alzheimer's in that memory is affected but not to the same extent as Alzheimer's. Thinking processes are disrupted and patients appear confused. Patients will spend more time thinking and problem-solving than previously. The symptoms can deteriorate slowly or quickly.

Vascular dementia patients will often also have or develop Alzheimer's disease.

Dementia With Lewy Bodies (DLB)/Lewy Body Dementia (LBD)

This is the second most common type of dementia. It is named after Frederich H. Lewy, a neurologist who was working in Dr. Alzheimer's laboratory when he isolated this particular abnormality of the brain.

It is difficult for a doctor to definitively diagnose this disease as these abnormalities can only be picked up during an autopsy. The doctor has to take into consideration the symptoms, some of which seem to be specific to this dementia.

The Lewy body is a mass of protein plaques that form in the brain. This protein, alpha-synuclein, is common in the brain but when these clumps form in the cortex of the brain, Lewy Body Dementia results. However, it must be noted that Alzheimer's patients frequently also have Lewy Body Disease.

Symptoms

Because this disease is difficult to diagnose physically, doctors rely on symptoms, many of which are symptoms of other types of dementia. Some of the symptoms are also indications of other diseases or conditions.

- **Hallucinations.** Although these do not belong to this disease alone. People with schizophrenia often hallucinate, as do drug abusers.

- **Tremors.** This symptom can also be found in diseases like Parkinson's.
- **Unusual sleep patterns and disturbances.** Also found in heart patients, Lewy Body Disease patients often complain of tiredness during the day. Their dreams can involve extreme physical activity like walking, running, or kicking.
- **Zoning out.** Patients will often seem to be not with the present moment, staring blankly into space, "zoning out." Everyone zones out occasionally due to boredom, stress, or grieving.
- **Mobility problems.** Problems with mobility are common with this disease, but as well as many other conditions also have this symptom. They will have balance problems and their movements will become slow and stiff.
- **Memory loss.** This is present here, as well as all other types of dementia.
- **Decision-making problems.** They will lose the ability to make decisions, as will patients with other classifications of dementia.

I hope you can sympathize with the doctor who is trying to give a name to your patient's disease. One of the factors peculiar to this disease is that the symptoms can change rapidly daily or even during one day. Another clue for the doctor is when the symptoms appear—with Lewy Body disease, mental issues occur before bodily issues.

The doctor may also pinpoint the disease through genetics. They may ask questions such as, "Have other family members had a similar condition?" and "What is the age of the patient, as this condition can start as early as 60 or as late as 85?"

Treatment

Once the doctor is convinced that they are treating Lewy Body Disease, they will be careful in prescribing any medication that may worsen the condition. Non-drug solutions need to be explored. Patients respond well to physical therapy and physical activities like stretching or balance exercises. Ballroom dancing could also be explored.

Mood enhancers can also be explored, like music, as these patients can have rapidly changing moods. It is a difficult disease for carers to deal with. A strong support group is advised. The carer will have to be aware of just what activity will help the mood of the patient in order to enhance their quality of life. Remember, this patient's mood and abilities could change frequently during the curse of a single day.

Parkinson's Disease Dementia

Parkinson's disease has been referred to in scientific studies since 175 A.D. when it was referred to as "shaking Palsy." It was recognized in Ayurvedic and Ancient Chinese medicine, but it was only in 1817 that Dr. James Parkinson wrote *An Essay on the Shaking Palsy* (News-Medical, 2019), giving the disease credence in the medical field. It was not until the 1960s that the chemical changes in a patient's brain were recognized as contributing to the degeneration of Parkinson's patients.

The clumps of alpha-synuclein that are found in other dementia types are also found in a Parkinson's patient's brain. The position of the clumps gives the definitive symptoms of each disease. In Parkinson's, the clumps are found in a deep area of the brain. The clumps set up the degeneration of the nerve cells. Parkinson's disease is not curable but treatments can help lessen the symptoms.

I need to stress that a Parkinson's diagnosis does not mean that the patient is headed for dementia, although a high percentage of patients will develop dementia in the later years of their life. If dementia develops, it will develop about 10 years after the initial diagnosis.

Symptoms

The disease and its symptoms get worse as time moves on. Several symptoms are similar to other degenerative diseases of the brain.

- **Tremors.** One of the first symptoms to be noticed; this might be tremors in the hands. But that is not definitive for Parkinson's alone. There are other reasons for tremors in the hands and limbs.
- **Slower movement.** Movement gets slower and you may notice that the way a person walks changes.

Because of the tremors and movement problems in general, things like handwriting change.

- **Posture and balance.** Also, due to tremors and movement problems, things like posture and balance will be affected.
- **Trouble sleeping.** Sleeping patterns will be disrupted.
- **Speech.** You will notice that speech begins to deteriorate.
- **Hallucinations.** The patient could become disoriented and hallucinations may be triggered.
- **Mood.** Irritability and depression are also common symptoms.

Treatment

Although Parkinson's is a degenerative disease, there are medications that will lessen the symptoms or even fully control the earlier symptoms. Patients could also try Deep Brain Stimulation surgery but, as with all surgery, there are risks (Dementia.org, n.d.).

There are some who choose the natural route. A healthier lifestyle will look at the patient's eating habits and they will be advised to cut out foodstuff that will accentuate their symptoms. Exercise is also good, like walking. There have been tests that prove that Ballroom dancing, particularly the Tango and the Waltz, has given a better quality of life for hours after the lesson (Alzheimer's Association, 2022). Balance and control were also improved.

Mixed Dementia

This occurs when the patient has more than one type of dementia. It is common to find that the Alzheimer patient also has vascular dementia but that is not the only combination that can be found.

Symptoms

Because there is little variety in symptoms of all dementia, it is difficult to diagnose which two (or more) diseases are involved.

Treatment

Once the specific dementias have been isolated, treatment plans for each can be tried. A healthy lifestyle is also indicated. Eating habits will be adapted. Alcohol and tobacco use is discouraged. Exercise will help, as will keeping up social contacts.

Clinical studies are focussing on whether having mixed dementia speeds up and worsens the symptoms. Scientists are also exploring the possibility that mixed dementia could hold the clue to curing or stalling all types of dementia (Alzheimer's Association, 2022).

Frontotemporal Dementia (FTD)

First referred to as Pick's disease, this disease affects the frontal part of the brain. This part controls judgment, emotions, planning, speech, and movement. Patients will either suffer changes to their personality or their ability to communicate will be affected.

Symptoms

Because of the area that is affected, you may find marked changes in personality. Symptoms could be:

- **Loss of inhibitions.** This means that they may disrobe in the most awkward places imaginable, for example.
- **Careless with words.** They will say what they wish, no matter where they are or who they are with. They will not realize when they are saying something hurtful as they lose all ability to be empathetic.
- **Poor hygiene.** They may forget to bathe. The caregiver will need to keep an eye on cleanliness and introduce it in a non-confrontational way.
- **Poor eating habits.** Their food preferences may undergo a change.
- **Lack of motivation.** They will lack the motivation to be up and doing.
- **Physical problems.** Their movements will become jerky, and they will have problems with balance.

Their limbs will be stiff and uncoordinated and they
might experience muscle spasms.
- **Verbal problems.** If their verbal ability is affected,
  you will find the following symptoms:
- Words will disappear as they are trying to converse
  and their thoughts will end up being incomplete.
- Their grammar may become jumbled to the point
  that their audience will not understand what they are
  trying to say.
- Their speech may become unclear or hesitant.
- They may be unable to comprehend or follow simple
  commands.

Treatment

The symptoms can be treated but the disease cannot. It is
incurable. The symptoms can be controlled or lessened using
several drugs. Treatments are indicated to improve the
quality of the affected person's life.

Huntington's Disease

This is a hereditary genetic disorder with symptoms similar
to Alzheimer's. The onset of the disease is likely to occur in
the patient's 30s but it can occur as late as their 50s. The
propensity for this disorder lies in one faulty gene.

George Huntington, M.D. gave his name to the disease in
1800 when he discovered what caused the symptoms of this
disease.

The abnormality of the gene interferes with the patient's ability to reason and move. The patient may be subjected to unplanned, involuntary movement.

Symptoms

There are some other symptoms that help with diagnosis. A neurologist will use the symptoms, scans, and genetic history to make a diagnosis.

The usual symptoms are:

- **Frustration.** Diminished thinking, concentration, reasoning, and memory lapses will lead to frustration in the patient in the early stages. It will affect the patient's ability to plan.
- **Speech problems.** The patient's speech will be affected.
- **Involuntary movements.** They could develop facial tics along with involuntary movements of all their limbs.
- **Behavioral changes.** Changes in their behaviors become marked. They could become irritated with things that they had just accepted before.
- **Mood changes.** Anxiety and depression could escalate.

Treatment

As with other dementias, the symptoms can be treated but the disease cannot. The disease will continue to degenerate and caregivers will need to give more and more support as the years progress.

Caregivers need to

- establish a good, almost rigid routine.
- help break down tasks so that they do not overwhelm the patient.
- anticipate and avoid situations that will upset the patient.
- make sure that the patient has outside stimuli and social interactions.

Creutzfeldt-Jakob Disease

The normal brain has folds but when a patient has Creutzfeldt-Jakob disease, abnormal folds develop in the brain, causing the onset of dementia. It happens quickly and worsens rapidly. It is a rare form of dementia and usually makes its appearance at 60 years old. It is strange because it can be genetic or just appear out of the blue. It could also, in a tiny proportion of cases, be due to an outside source, like eating meat from infected sources. Because of its similarities to mad cow disease, it has earned the nickname "human mad cow disease." It must be stressed, though, that there have been no cases of the bovine mad cow disease being passed on to humans.

Medical equipment can also transfer the diseased protein to the patient. Blood transfusions, harvested organs, and sperm donations from affected donors could also transfer the disease to the recipient.

Symptoms

The symptoms could be divided into mobility problems and conceptual problems.

- **Mobility problems.** Mobility problems could cause tics in various muscles of the body. The ability to walk will be compromised. Seizures may also occur. Their balance will be affected.
- **Conceptual problems.** Memory and concentration will be affected and worsen as the condition worsens. Mood swings, confusion, and depression are common. Most patients will not be able to get a good night's sleep.

Treatment

There is no cure for this disease but drugs may be prescribed to treat the symptoms.

Normal Pressure Hydrocephalus

This disease is typified by a buildup of fluid in the brain. It is sometimes possible to surgically insert a shunt to drain fluid into the stomach. Fluid in the brain is dangerous as it can damage the tissues alongside it. This treatment is successful in some patients but any damage that had already occurred cannot be healed.

The buildup of fluid in the brain can be the result of head trauma but sometimes the cause is unknown. All that is sure, in these cases, is that it will affect patients from the age of 60 onwards.

Symptoms

There are three definitive symptoms of normal pressure hydrocephalus:

- **Struggling with decision-making.** Thinking is slower and the patient loses the ability to plan ahead. They will also be almost incapable of making decisions.
- **Movement problems and tremors.** Their legs will be weak and they may experience tremors in their legs. When they walk, it will look as though they have sea legs as they seem to roll along with imaginary waves.

- **Incontinence.** They will lose control of their bladders and will need to wear incontinence underwear.

Other symptoms will be in alignment with many other dementia symptoms.

- They may experience bouts of nausea.
- Their vision and speech will be affected.
- Brain issues will include faulty memory, headaches, and a personality change.
- They will tend to be apathetic to their surroundings.
- Rapid mood changes are very likely.

Treatment

Once a doctor has been alerted to the possibility of the patient having this condition, they will rely on scans, lumbar punctures, and a physical examination in the doctor's room.

The pressure can be relieved by using the aforementioned shunt. Other than that, drugs will be used for the treatable symptoms. However, the brain damage will be irreversible.

Wernicke-Korsakoff Syndrome

This syndrome is almost always self-inflicted, as it is commonly found in alcoholics. It is caused by a severe shortage of vitamin B1. It consists of Wernicke encephalopathy, which causes brain damage. As these symptoms wane, the Korsakoff syndrome takes over and continues damaging the part of the brain dealing with memory.

This syndrome can also develop in AIDs and cancer patients.

Symptoms

Wernicke encephalopathy has the following symptoms:

- **Physical and movement problems.** Tremors occur along with a lack of muscle coordination in the lower limbs.
- **Eye problems.** Eye problems like battling to focus and moving abnormally.
- **Memory loss.** Loss of memory is a common symptom.
- **Hallucinations.** As with the other diseases we have discussed, hallucinating can occur.

When the Krosakoff syndrome takes over, permanent brain damage occurs and brings the following symptoms:

- memory issues
- making up stories to cover up the loss of memory
- hallucinations

Treatment

The symptoms may be treated but any brain damage that has occurred will be permanent.

Chronic Traumatic Encephalopathy (CTE)

Sportsmen, like boxers, who have received many knocks and injuries to the head, will possibly develop this condition years after they have left the sport. Each injury will affect some part of the brain and could lead to permanent brain injury. The power of the brain will degenerate as the years pass and could culminate in permanent dementia.

Symptoms

The continued abuse in the ring or on the field will cause the brain to degenerate slowly and the following symptoms will appear:

- **Memory loss.** Memory loss and confusion will be evident.
- **Impulsive behavior.** They tend to act impulsively and aggressively. They will be slow to acknowledge their part in their impulsive behavior.
- **Mood changes.** They will be prone to have fits of depression.

Treatment

As with other dementias, symptoms are treatable but damage is permanent.

REVERSIBLE OR NOT?

The above dementia types cause brain damage and are therefore irreversible but there are some types which, once medically treated, will reverse.

Delirium

Infections that lead to high fevers can cause a patient to become delirious. This delirium causes confusion in the patient. Once the fever subsides, the patient should return to normal. Care should be taken when an elderly person has an infection due to influenza or a UTI, as delirium could result.

When a patient has been on heavy drugs, either medical or recreational and they suddenly stop, withdrawal could cause delirium. This can also occur if the patient has an extreme reaction to the medication.

In some rare cases of a stroke, delirium could result.

Pernicious Anemia

Pernicious anemia is caused by a severe shortage of Vitamin B12. B12 is essential as it helps carry oxygen throughout the body. When the brain is deprived of oxygen, delirium can occur. It is treatable with B12 tablets or injections. Pernicious anemia can be hereditary or can occur due to autoimmune or stomach issues.

The symptoms of pernicious anemia include shortness of breath, tiredness, and dementia. Once the condition is treated, the symptoms should disappear. It may be necessary to take a B12 supplement for life.

Subdural Hematomas

These are blood clots in the brain that occur through some trauma, like a car accident. The elderly are more likely to develop blood clots in the brain from falls or loss of balance if they hit their heads. There is treatment available. Medication or mild surgery similar to an angiogram can be used to dissolve the clot.

Symptoms of a blood clot in the brain are similar to those of many of the dementia conditions.

Thyroid Disease

If the thyroid malfunctions, there are repercussions throughout the body, including the brain. More females have thyroid disease. The patient presents symptoms similar to dementia. It is easily controlled with medication that will be a life-long commitment.

Tumors

If the patient has dementia as a result of a tumor in the brain, they will display other symptoms totally unrelated to dementia symptoms like vomiting and headaches. When the tumor is treated the dementia symptoms will disappear.

Toxic Reactions to Drugs or Chemicals

The dementia that results from exposure to toxic products will disappear once the patient is removed from the area or from the offending drug.

Heavy metal poisoning and toxic chemicals could cause dementia-like symptoms. Lead has been removed from paint for this very reason. Examples of other toxic products are carbon monoxide and mercury.

Alcohol and drug abuse are also considered to be toxic to the brain. As long as the abuse has not led to brain damage, the dementia symptoms should disappear after complete rehabilitation.

THE SEVEN STAGES OF DEMENTIA

The global deterioration scale has established the seven stages of dementia to help doctors diagnose dementia patients. It is split into two parts, namely, pre-dementia and dementia stages.

Pre-dementia

This consists of three stages:

Stage 1: No Cognitive Decline

While the patient is in this stage, family, friends, and the patient themself are not aware of any changes in demeanor or ability.

Stage 2: Mild Cognitive Decline

Although this is not a definitive stage for dementia, as the changes are similar to what can occur with normal aging, it is hallmarked as the actual time when family and friends begin to be alerted to the fact that all might not be well. Forgetting names and words are features of this stage. At this stage, they may also start losing things as they forget where they have put them.

Dementia at this stage cannot be diagnosed but it also cannot completely be ruled out.

Stage 3: Mild Cognitive Impairment

Family and friends can look out for these signs if they are worried that their loved one is heading toward dementia:

- getting lost in familiar surroundings
- battling to concentrate and get the job done
- forgetting the names of family and friends
- reading without full comprehension

At this stage, the patient is aware of their forgetfulness which will lead to agitation.

Dementia Stages

The patient can be assessed for a positive diagnosis.

Stage 4: Mild Dementia

The patient becomes more aware of what is happening to them and is inclined to withdraw from social settings. They refuse to acknowledge what is happening to them. They will need a lot more help at this stage. They could become disoriented and have difficulty recalling events. They will also have difficulty in:

- managing their finances
- recognizing people

Stage 5: Moderate Dementia

At this stage, the patient may have difficulty remembering vital information like their home phone number or their address. They will need help with complex chores but will be able to take care of normal functions.

Stage 6:Moderately Severe Dementia

This is a distressing phase for family and close friends as the patient is likely to have forgotten who you are. They will forget what happened yesterday but will remember details from their past. They have a tendency to wander.

Stage 7: Severe Dementia

The brain ceases to make connections with the body. The patient will need help with all the normal activities, like feeding themselves. They may lose the power of speech as well.

WRAP UP

As can be seen, a doctor will have difficulty in diagnosing the dementia type just from the symptoms that patients display as many of the symptoms are similar. I liken their job to that of a detective, looking for clues and sifting through evidence.

Scans, genetics, and specific symptoms will all help with his diagnosis. A time frame will also help them come to the right decision. Some symptoms will help to steer them in the right direction, for example, loss of bladder control will steer them to normal pressure hydrocephalus. However, loss of bladder control can be aligned with other health issues as well. So do not be alarmed if it takes time and specialists to put a name to the dementia that your patient has. But in the end, treatment is going to be the same.

I hope this chapter has helped you understand that your loved one cannot help the symptoms they are displaying. In the next chapter, I will go over what you can expect to happen in the first three stages of dementia. After that, there will be chapters devoted to all the other stages as well.

STAGES 1–3 (PRE-DEMENTIA)

The detail in Chapter 1 helps the family and the main carer understand what they are dealing with. When the type of dementia is diagnosed, it helps the carer adjust the way that they deal with the patient. This chapter deals with the very beginning of the story.

The first three stages are defined as the early stages of dementia or pre-dementia. There Is no firm dividing line between the various stages. People are different and they may display symptoms in a different order to what is the norm. They will drift from one stage to the next, pulling in some, or maybe all, of the symptoms from the new stage.

The carer needs to be able to tell when the patient moves from the early stage to the middle stage so that they can adjust their care.

CHARACTERISTICS OF THE FIRST THREE STAGES

The first three stages are broken down as follows:

1. No cognitive decline
2. Age-associated memory impairment
3. Mild cognitive impairment

These three stages are similar to normal age-related problems. It gives the family time to see if there is actual dementia or if it is a condition that is treatable. So now may be the time to get the family member tested so you know what is in the future. Testing early is extremely important if there is a history of dementia in the family. It won't change the course of events but it will prepare everyone for the stages that follow.

If the family member shows signs of confusion and memory loss, early diagnosis and intervention can slow down the progression of the disease. It gives you the prime carer time to plan for the future. The people who need to be consulted for help could be:

- doctors
- counselors
- legal advisors
- financial advisors and
- family members.

Caring for a dementia patient can be debilitating for the carer if she doesn't have support. Do not be afraid to farm out some of the above responsibilities.

Stage 1

Everything appears normal as we cannot see what is happening to the brain without medical intervention. A scan may pick up the early signs. There is no need for a carer as the patient seems fully functional. There might be small memory lapses which could be put down to an age factor. The patient is able to work, drive, and fend for themselves. There is no time frame as it depends on the patient and on how they have looked after themselves previously and now.

Stage 2

The patient at this stage will be a bit more forgetful, but again, this is a normal sign of aging. Although the patient may still be employed, it might be found that they take a bit longer to do tasks but it will still be safe for them to drive, for example. The time frame is as for stage 1.

Stage 3

It starts to become apparent that all is not well with the patient. If they are driving, they may get disorientated and get lost. There will be problems with memory and work may not be the place for them anymore. They forget essential things and will find it hard to keep their concentration on the task at hand.

A proper clinical diagnosis is possible at this stage. Their family will be advised to start thinking about a carer. It might not be necessary to have a live-in carer at this stage as they will probably be able to take care of themselves as far as getting to bed and showering. If they live with family, night-time care will be overseen.

Tips for Preventing or Slowing Down Dementia

Dementia is caused by brain damage. It can escalate in some patients, and in others, it can be slow. There are some things that the carer can do to slow down the dementia. If the patient is just displaying aging symptoms, the following tips can help keep dementia at bay.

Lifestyle changes are important when caring for a patient who may be on the borderline of dementia. For instance, you, the carer, and your loved one can work on the following:

- Make sure that your loved one gets enough good quality sleep. A tired mind cannot think clearly.
- Both you and your loved one need to have a positive outlook. If they fumble, make light of it so that they don't get stressed about being clumsy. There is so much negativity in the world. There is no need for your loved one to dwell on horrific news like wars, famine, and riots. There is nothing your loved one can do to make the world a better place but you can make their world more comfortable and positive. If

they have been diagnosed with dementia, do not allow them to dwell on it, use any method you can to distract them from that disturbing diagnosis.

- Limit the use of alcohol or get them to give it up completely.
- If they are a smoker, help them to minimize the use of tobacco.
- Make sure that you both follow a healthy diet. You will need this as much as they do in the coming months. You need to be the best that you can be if you want to give your loved one the support they need.
- Make sure that your loved one keeps doctor's appointments and, if possible, sit in on the visit so that you can be up to date on any measures that you need to implement. And, of course, as their carer, you will ensure that they take all of their medication. During the doctor's visit, make sure that all the patient's concerns are addressed and that they are given tips on how to deal with the concerns.
- Do not let your loved one just sit or lie around. Find an activity that they enjoy and be there with them. If they enjoy bowls, ask them to teach you the elements of it. Take them for walks. The walk does not have to be strenuous; you can pause to admire the flowers or the view.
- Encourage your loved one to use their brain. If they enjoy sudoku, crosswords, or quizzes, encourage

them to keep up with them. If they have a computer operating Windows software, a plethora of games are available. A cell phone has many apps to keep the mind occupied, Nurdle for those who like numbers or Wordle for those who enjoy playing with words. Matching games are also very good. Jigsaw puzzles and board games will keep you both occupied and amused. You might as well make your sessions with them enjoyable.

PREPARE FOR A DEMENTIA FREE LIFE

While that is not possible for your patient, it is necessary for you to make what adaptations you can to lessen the impact on the patient and to make changes that will help you to evade the disease, if not permanently, at least to slow or delay the onset. This is particularly important if you have cases in your family.

There are certain things that are beyond your control for healthy living. Although most of us are doing what we can for our planet, there are still too many issues with water and air pollution. So let's move on to what you can do to help you and your patient.

Risk Factors

First and foremost, you need to do everything you can to keep both of you healthy. I know that is easier said than done in this post-Covid living. If you happen to catch a bug that is doing the rounds, take care of yourself so that you can more effectively take care of your loved one. Do not be shy to ask for help. You need to build up your strength and a few days in bed, knowing that someone else is covering for you.

If your loved one gets ill, wear a mask when you are in close quarters and boost yourself (and them) with plenty of liquids and Vitamin C.

Make sure that you both get plenty of oxygen into your system, as the brain requires oxygen to work efficiently. Stay away from stuffy environments; get fresh air into your home. Open the windows for a bit, even in cold weather.

Free-moving blood circulation is necessary for a healthy body as the blood transports nutrients throughout your body, so both of you need to practice good health measures.

- If you are a smoker, it is important that you really try to give it up. It pollutes the lungs as well as the air around you. Secondhand smoke is just as dangerous as actual smoking. If you are not a smoker, do not start and keep away from smoke-filled rooms.
- Alcohol can be taken in moderation but it is even better to abstain completely.
- Follow a healthy diet. Many dementia sites advocate the Mediterranean diet.
- Get (or keep) active. Find something that you enjoy and make sure that you practice it on a regular basis. Walking is a good exercise. It can be taken as slowly

as you like. If you walk slowly, there is an added advantage as you can appreciate the sounds and view around you. Yes, you need to take time to smell the roses! Exercise will also help your circulation.

- Be sociable. Find a club to belong to, or invite friends and family over for a fun evening. This is stimulating for you and for your charge.

- Be careful. A walking aid will help prevent falls which could be a major problem as you get older. When you are out walking, you could also offer your charge your arm for support. Just make sure you are strong enough not to tumble down with your loved one when they lose balance. It would be drastic if both of you ended up injured.

- Exercise your brain. A healthy brain needs to be challenged.

It is never too early for you, the carer, to start taking care of yourself. Dementia starts many years before the first signs but taking care of yourself from the age of 30 or 40 can decrease your risk immensely.

Most of the issues discussed above are aimed at you, the carer, even though most are good practices for everyone.

There are three risk factors that you cannot control:

- Every five years that you age after 65 increases your chance of getting dementia.

- It is a hereditary disease. If you carry the dementia gene, you are more prone to develop dementia.
- Women are more likely to suffer from dementia. The research figures may be skewed as women tend to live longer than men.

CAN I SELF-DIAGNOSE DEMENTIA?

There are signs that you, the carer, can use to determine if your charge needs to be medically assessed for dementia. But generally speaking, the symptoms of normal aging and the early stages of dementia can be confused. If you are in doubt, it is preferable to get a medical opinion.

Aging Versus Dementia Symptoms

- In normal aging, forgetting a word is no big deal, but if your loved one forgets words and their conversation is static with many pauses while they wrestle with what they are trying to say, take this as a serious indication that they need to see a doctor. If they are battling to understand what you are saying, that is another red flag. Sometimes dementia patients may call common objects like a fork by another name.
- Lapses of memory are common to both, but those who are aging normally will be able to recall what they were trying to remember and will even draw attention to it by saying something like, "I

remember what I wanted to say," but the dementia patient will not be able to do this recall. They may even deny they have a memory issue. Their short-term memory will be defective but things that happened many moons ago will usually be remembered.

- The dementia patient will have problems following directions and will often get lost traveling a route that should be familiar to them.
- If the patient was normally a person who enjoyed being with others and they suddenly no longer want to socialize, it is time for a diagnosis.
- Complex tasks will baffle the dementia patient, as will anything that involves problem-solving. They have lost logical thought. Problem-solving and complex tasks may take the aging person a bit longer than they used to, but they will get there in the end.
- The elderly are fully capable of planning functions or even just their lives but this task will be beyond the capabilities of the dementia patient.
- A dementia patient loses control of normal motor functions.
- A dementia patient may undergo personality changes, they may become more laid back or more strict, depending on what their personality type was before but a dementia patient displays disconcerting personality changes.

- Anxiety, agitation, and bouts of depression are common with dementia patients—if they have never had these afflictions before, it is a cause for concern.
- A dementia patient will lose sight of what is socially accepted. We have all heard stories of nude dementia patients found wandering the streets.
- A normal aging person does not look at people with suspicion but the dementia patient may start to distrust people who are close to them. It is also possible that they will start hallucinating.
- And finally, the dementia patient displays confusion and disorientation, even in familiar surroundings.

TREATMENT OPTIONS

While there is no cure for physical brain damage, there are medications that will help manage the symptoms. The earlier the disease is diagnosed, the better chance there is to find a treatment for the symptoms. Medication will also help to slow down the progress of the disease. This will help the patient have a better quality of life for longer.

Bear in mind that a General Practitioner may hand your case over to a neurologist, a gerontologist, or a psychiatrist as they have more experience in dealing with the condition.

Dementia is a condition that affects families, communities, and in the long run, the medical system, so research is ongoing to find medications that will slow down, or maybe even halt, the disease's progression. At the moment, many of the medications have unpleasant side effects like:

- nausea
- vertigo
- vomiting
- diarrhea
- slower heart rate

Available medications include:

- Cholinesterase inhibitors can be used to treat Lewy-body dementia and Alzheimer's disease. There is a chemical called acetylcholine in the brain that is responsible for maintaining certain functions like memory, learning, and muscle movements. In the two mentioned diseases, the chemical is broken down too rapidly, which causes memory lapse. The Cholinesterase inhibitors work by slowing this breakdown and thus slowing down the progress of the disease.
- Glutamate inhibitors prevent the harmful overproduction of glutamate that accompanies dementia. Glutamate sends messages from the brain —too much or too little cause health issues. Diseases like Alzheimer's, Parkinson's, and Huntington's are typified by an overproduction of glutamate. A

glutamate inhibitor will help to control an overproduction of glutamate.

- Antidepressants or antipsychotics will help control any mood swings that the patient may have. Depression, anxiety, and agitation are common ailments for dementia patients.

Because dementia is a problem that is increasing in the number of affected people, there is constant research to find answers. You may be able to sign the patient up for a clinical trial. Your doctor will be the best one to approach if you want your patient to take this route.

WHAT ABOUT ME?

You are important to your loved one. You need to become aware of the signs, symptoms, and progress of the disease. This is for both you and your loved one. If you do not understand where they are coming from, it can tear down any reserves of patience you may have. Dementia patients do need a calm, sensitive person to care for their needs. Without understanding, you may lose it when you have to deal with the same question or the same situation for the 50th time. But once you realize that it is the disease and not your loved one, things become a bit easier.

As your knowledge base grows, you may consider sharing your growing expertise. You could volunteer at a center (if it does not drag you away from essential time with your loved one). You could spread your knowledge by giving talks or writing a blog. You could help others in your social group who may be going through a similar situation. You could be a sounding board for their concerns. You could join a support group, and if there are none in your area, you could start one. Caring for a dementia patient can be a lonely job if you isolate yourself. You may have to convince others that there is no shame in dementia. People still want to hide mental issues from the outside world, unfortunately.

WHAT CAN I DO AS A FUTURE CAREGIVER?

In stages 1 to 3, there may have been no definitive diagnosis, but you know there is a strong possibility that your loved one is at the start of dementia. The question will arise, "Do we need a carer?" Unfortunately, you are it.

As mentioned above, mental issues are still regarded as something to hide behind closed doors but that is not going to get you the help that you will eventually need. Open the door to the conversation and include your loved one. Let them feel that they are not being shunted around. They are still very *compos mentis* and should be taken into the discussion.

At this stage, your loved one probably has not been diag-nosed but you have noticed some changes in them. And you want to prepare them for possible future diagnoses.

Maintain respect for your loved one's personhood and dignity—you are there to support, not dominate—lead, not coerce. Find out what they would prefer if things went bad. Would they want to stay where they are with a live-in carer or would they want to go to a facility where they will get help 24/7 if need be? Find out if they are prepared to move now before things get beyond you both. If they want to move a bit later, make sure that they have a hand in choosing his facility. The two of you could examine what facilities are available. Maybe even take a trip to view them. It may be necessary to put them on a waiting list. Chat with anyone you know who is living in a facility and ask them for pros and cons.

Legal issues need to be discussed.

- If there is no will, one needs to be made. A will can be made on an arbitrary piece of paper but it is better to get legal help to make sure that all bases have been covered.
- If there is a large estate, your loved one may need to get a financial advisor if they don't already have one.
- They need to nominate someone to act for them by getting power of attorney now while they are still capable. If it is left too long, lawyers and maybe the court will be involved and they may be made a ward of the court.
- Discuss the living will with them. Get their feelings on the matter and organize it if they are agreeable.

- Help them examine their options for long-term care insurance.
- Keep a note of any changes in the condition of your loved one so that you can keep the doctor up to date. HIPAA protects the patient's information from being shared without their consent. As your loved one is heading toward a time when you will have to hear and be able to access his details, you need to know what is needed in order for you to be able to access their information for their good.
- You need to keep up to date with research and new possible medications. Become a member of one of the dementia groups on their website or Facebook page. Register for newsletters. If you look just before the reference section of this book, you will see the available resources.
- Consider how your life will be impacted once your loved one reaches further stages that will require more time and effort from you. If you have a family, consider how it will affect them as well. Prepare them for what lies ahead. Be honest and upfront as they will also need to be prepared to say goodbye to the person they once knew and hello to the person who is left inside their body. Give them time to adjust and be prepared to answer or research any questions they may have.

One person you cannot forget about and one who needs care is you. If you are not looking after yourself, you will be of very little use to your loved one. Enlist the help of others, family, or friends. Take time out. Regard it as almost like a job. No one will be prepared to work for a boss all day, every day, without a break. But that is what your caring time will look like if you are not careful. Get someone to stand in for you at least one day a week. Treat yourself to whatever you need, a new hairdo, a night out with friends, time to lose yourself in that new book, or whatever gives you pleasure. You need to spoil yourself now and again.

Now is the time to gather the names of people who will be able to help. Do not try to go this alone unless you have no alternative. You can't pour from an empty cup! (Kelly, 2018). This is a tagline shared among caregivers. When you aren't at your best, you can't be an effective caregiver.

3

STAGE 4 (MILD DEMENTIA)

When the patient reaches this stage, they will be aware that things are not right even though they will battle to acknowledge it. The deterioration will be evident to family members and close friends. A definitive diagnosis is now possible. Everyone involved (including you, the caregiver) needs to understand what is happening to the patient and how to move forward and make plans for the future. There is still a vestige of logical thought in your loved one and they must be encouraged to share what they envisage for their future care. Please understand that this stage is frightening for them.

CHARACTERISTICS OF STAGE 4

This stage is usually described as early-stage dementia. Episodes where your loved one forgets what happened a short while ago increase. It doesn't matter how often you try to remind them of the event; they will steadfastly deny that it happened. For example, if they wanted to go shopping and you took them shopping, they would deny it and may use words like "Why do not you ever take me shopping?" It will take a lot of self-control on your part to be understanding of their situation. It is useless telling them that you took them earlier that day; they will deny it and get upset with you. Rather brush it off with something like, "I know, I have been so busy lately. Maybe we can try tomorrow."

Their concentration will fail them. Be understanding when they lose track of what you are saying. It is the disease, not them. They would concentrate harder if they could.

Because of the forgetfulness and the difficulty they have in concentrating, you will need to help them take care of essential financial matters. If you do not, essential services may be suspended because the account was not paid.

They can no longer be trusted behind the wheel of a car. Familiar places will appear strange to them and they will be confused as to their correct route. This will lead to them getting lost, which could place them in danger in this modern world of ours. They should also not be allowed the freedom to go walking by themselves for the same reason.

As their concentration levels decline, they will lose track of conversations in a social setting and this may result in them withdrawing more and more from socializing. They will also experience difficulty in talking fluently and their ideas may become confused as they battle to join in with the conversation.

This stage could last for up to four years but you could anticipate the patient lasting up to 20 years as they go through the other stages.

HOW IS DEMENTIA DIAGNOSED?

Doctors are working, not exactly in the dark, but definitely in the dusk. The only way to definitively diagnose dementia is after death with an autopsy of the brain, but there are symptoms, which, when lumped together, give a fairly accurate "working diagnosis" of dementia. There are several tests to evaluate the patient and eliminate other possible diagnoses:

- There are two cognitive tests—the General Practitioner Assessment of Cognition (GPCOG) and Mini-Cog. These tests consist of questions that are asked of the patient. An important test is to draw a clock face complete with numbers. The dementia patient will omit some numbers, or will jumble the order of the numbers, or will put numbers outside the circle, or will not space the numbers correctly.

- A neurological examination will include testing:
- physical movement, including reflexes, balance, coordination, muscle strength, and tone
- eye movement
- speech
- memory

The doctor may also request a brain scan (CT, MRI, EEG, or PET).

- He may request blood and urine samples for analysis.
- A psychiatric evaluation will establish if there are signs of depression, mood swings, or other mental health issues that may mimic dementia.

WHAT KINDS OF CHANGES WILL I SEE IN MY LOVED ONE?

This is a hard diagnosis for you and your loved one. They will often deny that there's anything wrong with them. They will say that the doctor is talking nonsense. This comes from either not comprehending what the doctor says or from fear of what lies ahead for them. Some patients will take comfort in having a diagnosis and will not worry too much about their mental stability at this stage. For you, the diagnosis will help you to arm yourself with as much knowledge as possible to make your job as a carer easier. I am doing my best in this book to fill up any holes you may have in your knowledge.

Socialization becomes more difficult and they may withdraw more from family and friends or social situations. This may be due to a hearing problem, so it is best to get that checked when doing the other medical checks. It is, though, more likely to be that the conversation is difficult to understand as the brain takes longer to assimilate what they hear. If they are part of a large crowd, they could become confused trying to follow the conversation. You can try to limit social gatherings to just a couple of people at a time.

Personality and behavioral changes will begin to occur. They could become moody and snap at you for little things. You will need to remind yourself that it is the disease and not the person. It might be difficult to control your reaction. If you snap back at them, you need to forgive yourself and not keep replaying the scenario in your head. I know that is easier said than done, but remember that in less than an hour, they will have forgotten about it. I am not minimizing your response, but if you snap now and again, let it go.

Depression or agitation are common symptoms of dementia. I found it best to distract my loved one with something pleasant, something that they enjoy. You might like to gather things together that can be used to diffuse these situations. They are of an age when photos were kept in albums, go through the albums, and ask questions. You may be surprised at the stories they can remember. They will enjoy the trip down memory lane.

The short term memory is severely affected. They will not remember that their son visited yesterday, for example, and will bewail the fact that they never see their son. No amount of telling them that their son visited yesterday will help the situation. They could well become annoyed with you for telling lies. Rather say something like, "You are right. I will ask him to come around tomorrow." This diffuses the situation and gives your loved one satisfaction that someone listens to them.

Sleep

Sleeping patterns may be disrupted. Your loved one is no longer as active as before but may need to rest in the afternoon. If the rest in the afternoon turns into a sleep, there may be problems getting to sleep at night, just when you need the rest as well. Fortunately, this condition will usually disappear as dementia moves into further stages. It might be useful to ask the doctor for a mild sleeping tablet for your loved one.

There are several reasons why a dementia patient has sleep issues.

- The part of the brain that recognizes the circadian rhythm may be damaged.
- They may be experiencing pain.

- They may get cramps or have restless leg syndrome.
- Medications may have sleep issues as a side effect.
- They may have sleep apnea.

So what can you do to solve these issues? Discuss the problem with their doctor. A physical examination may find a physical cause for the lack of sleep.

If there is no medical reason for this issue, then examine their environment. Is the room temperature comfortable? Is your loved one confused because you have moved them to a better situation? Is the room too light or too dark? All of these could disrupt their sleeping pattern.

If you want to try natural remedies:

- Take your loved one for one or two walks during the day. They may be restless due to inactivity, and this restlessness will disturb their sleep.
- Don't let them have a long sleep during the day.
- Cut out caffeine in the afternoon and evenings.
- Give them a small snack before bedtime.
- Give them a milky drink at night. If they don't like that, then try a cup of herbal tea before bed. Chamomile tea is calming.
- Give them a relaxing back rub.
- Play soft, restful music.

Hoarding

Your loved one may ferret stuff away and then forget where they have put things. They may even accuse the people around them of stealing their precious stuff.

Reasons for Hoarding

Hoarding is a common side effect of dementia. The person feels neglected even if you have just nipped out to the bathroom. This sense of being alone is interpreted as "There's no one to help me if bad people come here. So I must put my precious stuff in a place they won't look." This is especially true if they can remember friends, brothers, or sisters teasing them by taking away their stuff.

The dementia has chased some of their nearest and dearest away as they do not like to see the degradation. They have lost their freedom, their job, and their memory, so special care must be taken that they don't lose their precious belongings. So they hide them. Their failing memory will make them forget where they put things and they are quick to accuse the people around them of stealing.

Managing Hoarding

You need to help them find their lost stuff. This gets easier over time as you will learn where their favorite places are. Once, I found his gold watch wrapped in a handkerchief and stuffed in a shoe. The shoe was then squashed under a chest of drawers. And in the meantime, everyone was accused of stealing it. So you may need to be innovative in searching for the items.

They are often plagued with too much time on their hands. Get a box filled with odds and ends, like pens, crayons, beads, semi-precious stones, buttons, and so on. Sifting through the items will keep them busy for hours.

They will get confused quite easily, and if they forget where the bathroom or their bedroom is, they start to feel vulnerable and may start hiding their treasures.

Repetitions

Another feature of dementia patients is saying or doing the same thing over and over again. It can be exasperating for the carer to listen to the same stories and answer the same questions. They have no knowledge that they have been repeating themself and it is counterproductive if you show your exasperation.

Distracting them with a walk or a snack will pause those repetitions, but you won't have seen the end of them. There will be much tongue-biting on your part as you cannot tell them that you have heard it all before. It will just add to their confusion or they may lash out at you in anger.

Sometimes a dementia patient will do the same cycle of actions over and over again. This is an indication of their confusion and of their boredom. Have some activities at hand to distract them.

HOW IS MY ROLE AS A CAREGIVER CHANGING?

Up to now, you have just been there as a support person. Someone they could call on to help out. But now, your role becomes more meaningful as their memory and abilities start to fail. Whereas earlier, you acted as chauffeur, now and then, they will need you to get them to doctor's appointments, social visits, and shopping. It may be necessary for their safety to take away car keys or even to get rid of the car. If they are behind the wheel, they are just an accident waiting to happen. There are many other ways that your role will change and you will need to free up some more time to help them in many ways.

- As their confusion grows, they may even lose direction in the house. There are premade labels for doors to the bathroom, toilet, and kitchen already but some homemade ones could be used for the other rooms in the house.
- If they are still cooking, you will need to make sure that the food doesn't burn. When the cooking is over, just make a quick tour of the kitchen to make sure that the stove plates are off and the water is turned off.
- You will need to oversee paying bills. Try to get as many as possible automated. For the rest, use the banking app so that your traveling for financial reasons will be less. Your loved one may not take to

this kindly as many in that age group regarded the visit to the bank as an outing. They come from a time when banking was personal and you developed a personal relationship with one or more employees who would address you by name. There may be some resistance to the change.

- You will need to draw on your patience frequently. Your loved one is easily frustrated when they try to do things that they used to do. If you get upset with them, it will not help them complete the task, and they will likely become more upset than they were before. If you offer to help them, do not be upset if they get angry with you.

- During Covid, some stores set up delivery systems that they have kept. Each delivery may have a small fee attached but when you think of the time, petrol, and wear and tear on your car. It might be worthwhile to consider.

- If you decide to take your charge shopping, make sure that they and you have a shopping list. Their confusion will make them hone in on some easy or favorite items, some necessities will be forgotten, and you may end up with too many items that were not needed. Before getting to the checkout, check the trolley contents against the shopping list.

- When a new baby arrives home, they will be welcomed into a baby-proofed home. You need to now dementia-proof the home. Stairs are a hazard for the elderly with or without dementia. If you have the funds, install a chair lift. If not, make sure that your loved one has you close at hand to help. It may be necessary to consider moving them downstairs in a double-story house.

- Check the lighting and correct any poorly lit areas, as your loved one's eyesight and depth management may be faulty.
- Check loose boards or loose carpets. You may recover from a trip but your loved one will probably fall, which could result in a dangerous injury.
- Many patients and caregivers find brightly colored Post-it notes with simple written reminders or words of encouragement are effective ways to maintain some degree of independence.
- Do Google research for systems that could help you summon help when needed. Some companies have a remote device connected to your phone line. When the button on the device is activated, an automatic phone call brings a helper on the line. They know where you are without you having to say a thing and can summon emergency aid quickly. You do not even have to be in the same room as the phone. The device may be a panic button or it could be embedded in a necklace or a bracelet. The hardest thing will be to convince the patient to wear it at all times, even when they bathe, as many falls occur in the bathroom.

- Set up a family WhatsApp group to keep all informed of your loved ones' condition or emergency status. You should use this group (or generate another group) to call for help when you need it. I know you will probably be loath to "bother" people but you must get help when you need it.
- If you have not set up a power of attorney yet, do it now before the patient gets worse.
- If you are employed, let your boss know what your situation is and see if you can adjust your working hours more flexibly to fit in with when you are needed. Caring could become a full-time occupation, so you need your boss to be behind you. It is also more important to get a family backup system going.
- Write it down! If you are trying to keep a job going, as well as caring for your loved one and keeping personal appointments in line, you need a diary. An online one works for me but you may prefer a book.
- Do not overlook your own well-being as you focus more on your loved one; schedule time for yourself and the activities that nurture your well-being physically, emotionally, and socially.
- Seek out the support of other caregivers or survivors; there are numerous online groups if there are no active ones in your community. Check through local hospitals, councils on aging, Hospice, or senior centers. Facebook has several excellent

support groups; many allow you to post anonymously.

It is necessary to let your charge do whatever they can as long as it is safe. They still need you to acknowledge that their contribution is valuable. You need to enlist the help of other family members or even employ someone to take care of tasks that you do not have time for. Now is not the time to be too proud to ask for help. You need to avoid burnout. I really cannot emphasize this enough.

PITFALLS AND WARNING SIGNS

At the start of this stage, you can allow your loved one many freedoms because you want them to feel in control of their lives. This is fine but you need to be on the lookout for strange things. The patient in this stage could still manage to do quite a lot for themselves, but their condition is going to deteriorate, and you have to step in when things get too much for them.

Driving

They will still know the basics of driving as taught to them many years ago but their concentration level is less than it was then. They are also prone to confusion, particularly when there is a lot of traffic on the road. The lack of concentration coupled with confusion is a disaster waiting to happen. You may get a frantic phone call from them or maybe a stranger because

- they may have had a fender bender.
- they may have taken a wrong turn and got lost.
- they may have just crumbled and stopped driving in the middle of the road.

You can thank your lucky stars that it was not more serious; that they had enough presence of mind to contact you, but unfortunately for them, you will now have to stop their driving privileges. They can no longer be trusted on the road. You will be tempted to just come out and say, "That's it. No more driving for you." This is not going to work. You will be faced with stubbornness, anger, or frustration from them. You will need to approach the situation in another way. Something like "The next time you want to go shopping, let's make an outing of it. We can go somewhere for tea and cake." You know your loved one; you instinctively know what will work if you keep calm.

If that phone call doesn't come, keep a check on the car. Look for any bumps, dents, or scrapes to help you make the decision to stop his driving. Also, take note of how long the trip should be and how long it was. If it was too long, they might have gotten lost but finally found their way back home.

Another way you can assess if his driving is safe enough is to let them drive you somewhere. If you are continually pressing the imaginary brake on your side, it is time to stop them driving. If you do not feel safe on the road with them, they are no longer capable of driving.

Personality and Behaviour

You will find that your loved one is more irritable than before. They may also get cross quicker than before. They are probably feeling confused and their reaction is to protect themself. At this stage of dementia, their personality will quickly revert back to their normal self. But if there are sudden changes in personality or behavior, or if there is sudden confusion or slurred speech, this may indicate another health condition. Seek medical help immediately to check for stroke, injury, infection, or other causes.

Serious changes in personality and behavior will take a while to be noticeable and will be evident in the later stages of dementia.

Medication

At this stage, they should be capable of managing their medications themselves but there may be periods of forgetfulness when essential medication is not taken. If you do not already have one, get a pill box for the week for morning and evening medication. You may have to take on the weekly job of filling the container for the next week. I made it a social occasion. I visited, we put on his favorite program on the TV and chatted and watched while I prepared the week's medications. As we didn't live together at this stage, I phoned each morning to remind him to take his tablets and each evening, I popped around to chat and medicate. If you live together, it is much easier to supervise the medication. If they are not supervised, even at this stage, they may forget to take their tablets. Or they could take them, forget that they took them, and take them again. Over or under-medicating is a very real problem if left unsupervised.

Conversations to Avoid

A dementia patient can be very sensitive about their condition. The following conversations should be avoided:

- Do not correct them. If they are wrong about something, let it slide. If you correct them, you may
- make them angry or
- embarrass them.

And you will have achieved nothing. The statement will not be corrected and they will forget what they originally said.

- Arguments. They are in no fit mental state to defend their views. It is not important that you or they are right. Instead of calling them out, change the subject to a pleasanter one.
- Jog their memory. If they have no memory of something, no amount of pushing them to remember

is going to work. The end result will be that you are both frustrated and maybe angry.

- If they ask when a deceased loved one is coming home, do not tell them that they won't be coming home because they are dead. The dementia patient will have no memory of the loss and you do not want them to grieve all over again.
- Get to know which topics can be discussed and which must be left alone (Marley, 2013).

SOME TIPS

These tips will help you cope with your loved one:

- Set up a daily routine. This way, they will acclimate to the changes from one activity to the next.
- Never bombard them with many instructions or conversation topics at a time. Keep to one item at a time. Too much at a time will confuse them.
- When in their company, use humor as much as you can. This will help keep you focused on them. Focus on interpreting his feelings, wants, and needs.
- Don't get angry or annoyed in front of them. They will not understand your frustrations. They will just end up more confused than before. If you need to gather yourself, you can leave the room for a few moments to stabilize your emotions.

- Do not try to rationalize things. They will not understand the logic. You cannot argue with them. Just bite your tongue, count to 10, and smile!
- If they are restless, take them for a walk. Get them dancing or singing. Play their favorite tunes.
- Get them to help you around the house. Choose simple tasks similar to what a 10-year-old could handle (National Institute on Aging, 2019).

WHAT SHOULD WE PREPARE FOR NEXT?

I hope the hints and tips in this chapter will help you get through Stage 4. Rest as much as you can during this stage and try to clear out anything that you have been putting off due to lack of motivation. As your loved one enters the next stages, you will be giving up much more of your free time, so if you have not got your support team sorted, do it now. You will need help.

There will be a deterioration in your loved one's condition, abilities, and quality of life. You will need to be much more hands-on in your care of the patient. If they live alone, you will have to rectify this. Either move in, get them to move in with you, or look for a place where they will get the care that they need. You will probably be ramming yourself up against a brick wall if you try to move them but you really need to be the decision maker now.

4

STAGE 5 (MODERATE DEMENTIA)

T hings will start to get a bit more difficult for the caregiver as the patient enters this phase. It is also a bad time for the patient, as their frustration at their inability to function normally grows. They will have problems doing tasks like dressing or buttoning shirts, and unfortunately, they will be aware of the problem. It is probably the worst phase for both the carer and the patient. The carer needs to be more hands-on, and the patient has to accept that there is going to be a need to depend on others a bit more.

As with all the phases, the transition to this phase will not be clear-cut. Some of the changes will start to appear toward the end of Stage 4 and some may only appear in Stage 6.

STAGE 5'S IMPACT

As the patient sinks further into Stage 5, they will need to be reminded (and eventually helped) to bathe and change soiled clothing. It is quite common for them to want to wear the same clothes for many days. It is probably because that is the easy way out. It requires no thought or decision-making on their behalf. It is up to the carer to address this in a pleasant way, such as:

- "Why don't you wear this dress today? I really like you in this."
- "This blue shirt makes your eyes pop! Let's change into it and give us all a treat when we see your eyes shining bright."
- "We are going to the shops today, so let's glam up and change into something special."

If you make the suggestion into a compliment, you are less likely to get uphill from them. The worst thing you could do is to tell them their clothes are dirty and must be changed.

Another problem with clothing is that the patient cannot make decisions according to the weather. In searing heat, they may be wearing a jersey and in cold weather, they are likely to dress in summer clothes.

FROM INDEPENDENCE TO DEPENDENCE

While it is helpful for the carer to assist with grooming, there are times when it is essential for the carer to take over. These are the times when it is no longer safe for your loved one to be left to their own devices.

They will start to have bouts of failing to get to the toilet on time, or they may even ignore the surge for a toilet visit.

WALK-ABOUTS

The exits need to be secured to limit your loved one, as they will attempt to wander off. This wanderlust is inherent in this condition. Whenever they are outside, the carer needs to be with them. Their sense of direction is disrupted and they get lost very easily. They are capable of walking miles. Their confusion will escalate and when found, they may be hard-pressed to give any personal information. Their safety is compromised when they go walkabout. They are an accident waiting to happen as they have probably forgotten to look in both directions before crossing a road. They are also targets for mugging.

DRIVING

This may be the time when family or carers step in with white lies. The patient may remember how to drive a car, but their perceptions are compromised, and once again, they are an accident waiting to happen. Their inability to judge distances could end in a rear-end collision. They may be confused by the colors of the traffic lights, when to go, and when to stop. They will more than likely confuse left and right turns, which will end up with them getting lost, hopefully in a good neighborhood; otherwise, their safety will once again be compromised.

Because their manual dexterity will start to fail, they will forget which hand or foot to use while driving.

So back to the white lies that you may be forced to tell:

- "I noticed that your car was making a funny noise. Can I take it for a spin?" When you get back, you can report that it sounds serious and needs to be looked at by a mechanic. You can then report that the repair is a major repair and the recommendation is to sell the car as it has reached the end of its life cycle with them.
- "Have you seen the damage on the passenger's side of your car? It is quite bad. I will take it to the panel beaters for you." Then continue to bypass their queries until they hopefully forget about it.

You will need to be innovative for your loved one's safety.

COOKING

We have all had little cooking accidents but a patient with dementia will put a pot on the stove and forget about it. It would be a plus if they actually had anything in the pot before setting the heat. While this will quickly result in damaged cookware, it could also lead to a fire which the patient will be incapable of suppressing. They may no longer enjoy foods that were once their favorite.

MEMORY

There will be a significant change in what they remember. Something that happened a few minutes ago may be forgotten but something that happened when they were a child will be remembered.

You may have taken them out to a special place yesterday, for example, to a favorite restaurant. Today they will say, "It has been so long since we went to that favorite restaurant of mine." Guard your tongue, but if you slip up and say, "But we went yesterday." they will argue that you didn't. Accept this gracefully and say something like, "Oops, sorry, my mistake." If you try to argue with them, both of you will end up frustrated. It is far easier to accept the blame.

It is frustrating for a caregiver to handle this, particularly if the patient is a loved one. There needs to be much biting of the tongue when they can't remember things. The carer needs to remember that it is the condition and not the person. The person cannot help themselves, so it is counter-productive to get annoyed with them. The easiest route is to agree with them and move on. As mentioned earlier, it will be helpful to bring out any photograph albums that the person may have and go through it with them. Ask them about the people, the place, and the situation. It gives them great joy to remember things.

Do not get upset when they confuse you with someone else. They may even think that you are their parent. Go with it no matter how hard it is; just remind yourself that they are not doing it on purpose; they can't help themselves. Be gentle and tell them that you love them. If they can't remember who you are, gently tell them about your relationship. Make sure that visitors are aware of this. It might be an idea to say something like, "Look who's come to visit! It's Sarah, your niece." This lets everyone off the hook.

They will frequently lose the thread of what they are saying, so conversations become sluggish as the person tries to recall a word or even their train of thought. Do not try to hurry them on or finish the sentence for them. If they say, "Now, where was I?" They have given you permission to intervene so you can help out.

Their memory is fractured and there will be some patching of their thoughts to try to make the thought a cohesive whole. This may entail them entwining other memories, which makes the story confusing to follow. You may feel that they are fabricating the story as it doesn't piece together. But be careful of addressing the issue. They are trying to overcome this memory lapse in any way possible. Do not argue with them, as this will end up with both of you being upset.

Let them talk about the past. They will remember details that will surprise you as you learn about their early life. Photos may help jog their memory. This will put them in a happy place.

PERSONALITY

During this stage, you will start to see changes in their personality. Changes in mood may happen quite quickly. Some mood changes may not have previously been a personality trait of theirs. Accept them for who they are now, and do not try to compare them with who they were. Unfortunately, that other person no longer exists and just as they may have to relearn who you are, you need to relearn and accept them for who they are now.

As mentioned before they tend to become suspicious of everyone. They put things in a "special" place and then forget where it is and will accuse the carer of stealing.

Things that they used to enjoy, like humor, may make them angry. They may be prone to sink into depression. They may experience other emotional changes, like being fearful of things that never bothered them before.

They may start to swear or indulge in inappropriate remarks and behavior.

TAKING CHARGE

Your duties will now start to encapsulate all aspects of your loved one's care. You have taken care of their bills and their personal needs. They will soon need to have all financial decisions taken away from them. To do this, you need a power of attorney. If you have not already got that in line, this stage is the last stage you will get cooperation from the patient. If you leave this to stage 6, they are incapable of making decisions, and you may have to make them a ward of the court for their financial protection and yours.

Power of Attorney

A power of attorney (POA) is a legal document granting a trusted person certain rights and decision-making abilities when an adult cannot make these decisions for themselves. If you do not have a power of attorney, you will not be able to make certain crucial decisions. It is a legal document and it is preferable that a lawyer sets it up. With our modern lifestyle, there are many forms available online. It is fine if the family wants to go this route as long as they are aware that there may be pitfalls along the way.

Let's look at some definitions of these legal documents to make this section clear:

- The title of *attorney* is given to the person who takes on the responsibilities listed in a power of attorney. This title is different from the attorney who works in the legal field.
- The person who is giving over the power of attorney is known as the *donor*.
- *Lasting power of attorney* (it used to be known as enduring power of attorney) enables a designated person (the attorney) to take care of financial concerns till the end of life of the patient (the donor).
- *Ordinary power of attorney* will only last as long as the donor feels it is needed.
- *Health power of attorney* exists to give the attorney the right to make legal decisions for the donor.

Lasting Power of Attorney

The lasting power of attorney (LPA) comes into effect as soon as it is registered. It needs to be set in place while the donor is still in a relatively stable state of mind. It usually comes into effect when the donor is no longer capable of making their own decisions in these regards.

Lasting Power of Attorney (Property and Financial)

This LPA gives full power to the attorney regarding financial and property management. They can buy or sell property in the donor's name. They can organize essential repairs or upgrades to the property. They can be held responsible for paying accounts and mortgages. They are able to invest money or cash in investments on behalf of the donor.

Lasting Power of Attorney (Health and Welfare)

It is essential that the donor set this up while they still have mental stability. It must be signed by someone who knows them well and can attest to his mental acuity at the time of signing. It comes into effect when the donor can no longer make decisions themself. It covers

- necessary medical care.
- decisions regarding daily welfare like food and clothing.
- appointing a carer.
- choosing a residence when the patient can no longer care for themself.

"Living Will"

This document should be generated by the patient well before stage 4 dementia. However, it is not too late to get it done now. This is a document that gives the patient control over end-of-life decisions. It can include a do not resuscitate (DNR) order which hospitals are bound to abide by. It should be housed with the patient's doctor as well as the carer, whether that carer is at their residential home or an employee at the home where the patient now lives.

This document ensures that the patient's family is not faced with the decision of "pulling the plug." It will only be used if there is no hope for the patient's recovery, even if resuscitated.

The document could also be used in the case of organ donation.

It must be stressed that all the above documents should have been dealt with before the patient enters stage 5.

HOME CARE OR RESIDENTIAL CARE FACILITY?

This is probably going to be the hardest decision you will have to make. The patient can no longer live alone and care will be needed 24/7. You have a few choices.

Move In With Them

This is easiest for the patient. They will be in familiar surroundings. This is important for them as they can still move around and a sense of confusion is lessened when everything around them is familiar.

As this stage can last for more than a year, it is not a temporary solution. You will have uprooted yourself and lost your freedom. You will have to give up your job and a job is what defines many people. You will have left all your comforts behind. Maintaining a social life will be difficult.

Move the Patient in With You

You may think this will be easier but you will still be on call 24/7. Your job may still have to go, as will your social life.

Your loved one may be confused, even if they have visited your home on numerous occasions. They won't know how to get to the bathroom and kitchen, which could lead to stress on his side. If you furnish their room with familiar things, it may lessen the confusion.

If you share your home with a partner and children, you must consider the impact on their lives as well. As your loved one's condition deteriorates, your entire household will feel increased stress.

Get a Live-In Carer

It will cost a bit but your freedom to carry on with your job and social life is worth it. Your loved one will be in their home with familiar things but may possibly object to a stranger being in their home. You will still need to do checks on them. At first, you can pop in every day to assure them that you have not forgotten them. Then you can space the visits out once you are satisfied that all is the best it could be under the circumstances.

Residential Care Facility

If I am going to be totally honest with you, this will have to be considered as the dementia increases. So why not move early on when they can understand the situation? They will have time to get used to their new surroundings and every part of their daily routine will be supervised.

They will have periods when they kick at the solution you provided but that is going to happen no matter what solution you try.

There are cons to this solution. These places are expensive. And you will probably find that the patient's medical care insurance does not cover this. If you are wealthy, you won't have a problem with the added expense. If you are on the bread line, the government will step in to help. But if you are a normal middle class daily, this may not be a possible solution for you. Financial considerations and how to choose a facility will be discussed further in Chapter 5.

Guilt

No matter what you decide, you will have feelings of guilt and a sense of having failed a loved one. Friends and family may have you second-guessing yourself as to what you have decided. And there is still a need for the caregiver to monitor the patient's well-being as their guardian, advocate, or as the one holding their POA/Healthcare POA.

A CAREGIVER'S CHANGING ROLE

As time progresses, your loved one's personality undergoes more changes until you feel that they are a stranger and not the person you looked up to for so many years. It might be worthwhile to remind you that as the days go by and your loved one's memory fails more and more, you are becoming a stranger to them. Try not to get upset if you have to reintroduce yourself or any other family members.

They are going to need more of your time as you will need to do more things for them. The job of a carer is going to become a full-time one. Their increasingly limited abilities need you to be on the lookout for potential factors that could harm them. You may need to consider giving up your day job. That will be hard for many reasons.

- If you worked for the same company for years, the chances are you received promotions. You will be lucky if they take you back after a sabbatical lasting a few years. If you have to look for another job when your full-time care is over, you will probably have to start over with a new company.
- You will need to ask yourself if you can financially manage if you are without a job for a few years. The loss of income could bring other stresses to the fore. There will also be increased household expenses.
- Your housekeeping chores will escalate as you deal with an incontinent patient.

There will be an added strain on you if you are trying to run two homes: your loved ones and yours. The risk of burnout is very real and you need to safeguard yourself against it. You will be useless as a caregiver if you start to need care yourself.

- The first step is to get back up. It doesn't matter how strong you feel you are; you cannot do this alone. See if there is any family member who would give up some time, hopefully on a weekly basis. If that is not possible, look for support groups who may be able to help you. If you belong to a religious community, appeal to the congregation for help. Now is not the time to be proud. If a full-time carer does not fit your pocket, investigate if you can get a carer for a day a week. Many towns now offer an adult daycare solution.
- If you manage to get some time off, do not waste it on household chores. Do something for yourself, something that gives you pleasure. Some suggestions are:
- Go for a walk in the garden or around the block.
- Take a long relaxing bath. Pop some aromatherapy bath salts in and lie back with a glass of wine or cup of tea or coffee.
- Listen to music while going about your chores or on your walk.
- Listen to a favorite podcast.
- Indulge yourself with a treat.
- Sit outside with a good book for half an hour.

- Look after your health. Do not just grab chips or sweets because you do not have time to stop and eat a decent meal. There is always time for good healthy food and snacks. It is just a matter of organization. If you get sick, it is an added stress on you, the home, and the patient.
- You need to get enough uninterrupted sleep. If your charge requires attention at night, you need to enlist some help (as mentioned earlier).
- Keep hydrated with water in preference to tea or coffee. Water-rich fruits like melon, strawberries, and peaches can be eaten as snacks or as desserts.
- A pet can help calm down your charge—but only if they like the pet. They may rebel against a new pet but love to cuddle with an established pet.
- Get them to help you around the house, giving them tasks similar to what you would expect a child to handle. They need stimulation to try to slow down the degradation of their brain.
- Keep them occupied with
- large-piece jigsaw puzzles.
- coloring—buy yourself an adult coloring book and get them a child's coloring book and sit together chatting while you color.
- dancing to their favorite music
- crafting—buy a blank page scrapbook and together select pictures to paste into the book. You may have

to do all the cutting but they should manage to glue the pictures in with some help.

- making an album of their photos or postcards from places they have visited.
- encouraging their artistic talents with play dough.
- building up a memory box full of treasures from their past or buying some new things.

WARNING SIGNS AND PITFALLS

Family and friends who have not been involved with the day-by-day care may be startled by the deterioration of your loved one's memory. They may feel hurt if they don't remember them or think they are someone else. You will, of course, keep them up to date on their condition but seeing it in real time will be disconcerting to some. They may retreat and be unwilling to visit again and will definitely not be prepared to help out.

This lack of understanding and support may hurt your feelings but will almost certainly add to the stresses you are feeling and experiencing. The more you try to do, the closer to exhaustion you become. Exhaustion leads to burn out, which causes you to isolate yourself from people who could help keep your spirits up. The lack of support that you get will frustrate and anger you and could lead you to depression. Your health and well-being will directly impact the patient. Do not forget yourself.

The Patient

As the stage progresses, your loved one will have increasing difficulty with speech. They may not be able to let you know when they are in pain or have injured themselves. You will have to be observant and watch out for small signs like cringing when they use their hands, limping when they walk, or rubbing a body part.

There will be physiological changes in their body. They will lose control of bodily functions and will have to wear incontinence underwear. If there is continuous leaking, it may set up a urinary tract infection. They may not be able to tell that it hurts, so you will need to be observant. If unattended, the infection could lead to delirium, which could be put down to the dementia rather than to something wrong with the patient.

You need to keep a lookout for skin infections, eczema, insect bites, and chafing. Make sure that you treat anything on the skin and generally keep the skin moisturized. After a bath or shower, make sure that the skin is properly dried. On hot days, keep the skin cool by passing a cool cloth over the face, hands, and wrists.

The body will lose its capability to distinguish between hot and cold. They may put on a heavy jersey on hot days or wear next to nothing on cold days. This could put them in a dangerous situation. For example, they may hold their hand under a scalding hot tap and suffer painful burns or clutch onto a metal pole with their bare hands when it is snowing outside. I know that these two are extreme situations but they could happen.

Their taste buds will change and what they once enjoyed may be distasteful. Their appetite will decrease as well. Here are some tips to make mealtimes enjoyable and healthy:

- Make everything on the plate bite-sized and do not be uptight if they choose to use their fingers instead of implements. As their physical condition deteriorates, handling knives and forks could get difficult.
- Set up smaller meals four or five times a day.
- Food comes in many colors. Make their plate as colorful as possible. They say you eat with your eyes (Nuush, 2020). Decorate the table with colors as well —colorful serviettes, placemats, flowers, and so on.
- Do not let them eat alone. Make up a plate for yourself and chat while you eat.
- Make mealtimes social times.

Your loved one is going to need help dressing as their mobility will impact their ability to do up zippers and buttons. You may have to get rid of all clothing that requires finger manipulation and buy:

- Pants with elastic waists and no zips or buttons.
- Tee shirts or jumpers that pull on.

- Shoes that are pull-on or have velcro fastenings. Laces and buckles will be too hard to manage. Make sure that the shoes have good, non-slip soles.
- Natural rather than synthetic fibers. Natural fibers can breathe and keep the body at a more constant temperature.

WHAT NEXT?

Physical and mental changes continue to escalate. They will need more help doing everything from bathing, getting dressed, eating, and entertaining themselves. You are going to be pushed to your limit if you do not set up some assistance.

EASING THE BURDEN

"Caregiving often calls us to lean into love we didn't know possible."

— *TIA WALKER*

Do you remember what my friend said to me about his dad's dementia diagnosis? For three years he was angry with his dad, for three years he was angry with God, and for three years he was angry with himself. That's nine years of anger... alongside all the stress and sadness that also comes with being a caregiver.

I've never gotten those words out of my head. It rang true for me at the time, and all the while my mom and I were caring for my dad, I had to make a conscious effort to let go of that anger. It became important to me to do what I could to help other caregivers through this incredibly difficult time... because when you know what it's like, you can't bear to think of anyone else having to go through that without support.

I know you know that too... and although I'm aware that you have a ton on your plate right now, I'd like to ask for your help in reaching this support out to more people. The good news is that this won't take more than a couple of minutes, and it can easily be done while you're reading – you don't need to carve out any extra time. Showing other people where they can find this support is as simple as leaving a review.

By leaving a review of this book on Amazon, you'll show other caregivers where they can find supportive and empathetic guidance that will help them through this heartbreaking phase of their lives.

Simply by letting other readers know how this book has helped you and what they'll find inside, you'll show them that they don't have to go through this alone – and you'll point them in the direction of the guidance they need to get themselves through without burning out.

Thank you so much for your support. Caregiving can feel terribly isolating, and together, we can help ease the burden a little.

Scan the QR code to leave a review on Amazon!

STAGE 6 (MODERATELY SEVERE DEMENTIA)

If you are still the sole caregiver, you are in for a rough ride. It is more important now to get help to ensure your own health and well-being. Your charge is going to need a lot more of your time from now on, so you need to form a caregiving team.

You will feel that you hardly recognize your loved one as changes will now occur quite rapidly. They are bewildered by the change and can become very anxious. This anxiety could lead to obnoxious behavior where they are quick to anger. They will develop a resistance to bathing as their sense of hygiene has diminished greatly. They will soon lose their ability to recognize cues to go to the bathroom. They will not understand why hygiene, like hand washing, is necessary. They will no longer be able to figure out if they are hot or cold. You will have to monitor their clothing for the day.

You will be stepping in to help and supervise much more during this stage and burnout is a real possibility. As the carer, you may also start to feel that you are inadequate for the task of caring for them. You may also feel a sense of extreme failure.

CHARACTERISTICS OF STAGE 6

Increased dementia will affect the patient physically, emotionally, and mentally.

What Changes Can I Expect to See?

Your loved one will need help with eating as they will no longer be able to manage utensils. To make feeding easier, solid food must be cut into bite-size pieces. Potatoes and pumpkin-like squashes can be mashed. Try to limit solid foods as they may develop problems chewing and swallowing. Make sure that their plate is attractive with a healthy food balance.

Their personal hygiene will have to be taken care of by you and/or the team. You will need to help them shower or bathe. When toweling off, make sure all body parts are dry and moisturize their skin before helping them dress. Dressing will also need assistance as they will not know which item goes where. They are likely to put a vest over their shirt or underpants on top of their trousers. You will have got rid of the complex fasteners that clothing has and all their clothing should be of a pull-on or pull-up nature.

As dementia takes more of their brain, they will battle to verbalize what they want or what they need. Words will be random and they will find it hard to form sentences. Frustration at their inabilities will often lead to anger. This may never have been a part of their personality but you will notice other changes of personality until you won't recognize the stranger inhabiting your charge's body.

By now, you are used to their short-term memory being non-existent but their long-term memory will now start to disappear. Facial recognition fades and they will not recognize friends and family members. They may see a resemblance in family members and will mistake a loved son for a nephew or cousin or maybe even maybe their father. A hard day for you will be the day they don't recognize you, their primary caregiver. You will have to keep on reminding yourself that it is the disease, not the person.

Do you remember seeing videos of animals (or a child) seeing themselves for the first time in a mirror? They were confused and wondered where that strange thing had come from. The dementia patient is also confused by mirrors and will not recognize themself. They will be convinced that a stranger has entered the house. They will not understand the pictures and noises from a television.

Your loved one's circadian rhythm will be upset and they can no longer distinguish when to go to bed and when to get up. Because of this upset in the natural rhythm of the day, they may have trouble sleeping and will tend to wander at all times of the day or night. There is no solid reason for their wanderlust but many scientists believe that the patient may be trying to go home (even though they were home), go to work, or go shopping. It may also be because they are anxious and agitated. When you take them out, keep an eye on them and never leave them in the car alone, even if you know you will only be a minute.

Where you once identified a person who took life firmly in their stride with no time for nonsense, they now may appear as a frightened child when delusions and hallucinations invade them. These could lead to severe anxiety. The anxiety could escalate dementia. There may be times when they zone out, followed by periods of anxiety or violent outbursts.

They may have periods in the late afternoon when they become overly anxious, their behavior deteriorates, and they become agitated. This is called sundowning. Although there is no precise diagnosis for this trend, it is thought it may be a consequence of tiredness.

Movement becomes more difficult and they will battle to retain balance while walking.

Their sense of insecurity grows and they are likely to latch on to you as a haven in their ever-changing world. They will follow you as you go about your daily tasks. This is termed shadowing.

They will no longer have a sense of hygiene, being prepared to wear dirty clothes every day should you allow it. Their incontinence will increase as they no longer recognize their body's bathroom signals.

Stage 6 is called severe cognitive decline, so we can expect everything that has been going downhill to continue further down the track, and you will be in for some new deterioration as well. They are going to start to find basic tasks difficult.

Wandering

This has been discussed earlier, but in Stage 6, it becomes a real problem. They will wander off at the drop of a hat. If you question them as to why this happened, they no longer have the verbal power or the memory to tell you. Their safety is compromised when they wander off. There is a certain sector of humanity that enjoys being nasty to the weak and vulnerable.

Make sure that you, the carer, know what they are wearing before they take off. That shouldn't be too hard as you would have assisted them in getting ready. Inform your neighbors and the police to keep an eye open for them.

Reasons for Wandering

Some of the possible reasons that a dementia patient may wander if they have moved residence is that they want to go home, so they try to find their way. Their memories and their past are not in the new place. They may want to find their life again.

They could have had a memory of when they were employed and they want to get back to their job. They could also be searching for places that they went to when young.

They may have built up some excess energy and walking gets rid of it. They could also feel bored and walking was a habit that they did when they were bored, anxious, or angry.

Managing Wandering

You will need to try to establish why they wander. What set of circumstances happened before they took off? What was their state of mind? Were they anxious, depressed, or frightened? Were they trying to avoid a person?

Get them to the doctor as soon as possible to rule out any health issues or medication side effects. Observe if they appear confused after taking medication.

While you are going to do everything in your power to prevent them from taking off, you would be wise to take some precautions. They will no longer be able to tell anyone where they live or what phone number will alert the family. Make sure that they always have some form of identification, complete with their home address and your telephone number.

HOW IS MY ROLE AS A CAREGIVER CHANGING?

You will have to be more focused on your charge as wandering and shadowing become more frequent. If you take them out in the car, you cannot just run into a shop, leaving them in the car. They will get out and wander off when something catches their eye. They will not think of the implications. Somehow or other, the dementia patient has incredible walking power. They have been known to cover several miles.

With shadowing, you will need to be aware of them behind you all the time. A sudden turn or change of direction could end up in a collision. If their balance is at all off, they could wobble and fall, hopefully not doing any physical damage but they may become quite verbal.

If they are still at home, either their place or yours, there could be repercussions for everyone else who lives in the house. Your loved one will have no respect for the privacy of everyone else living in the house. This could lead to altercations within the family unit. Certain family members (spouse or children) could resent the amount of time you spend with your loved one. This will all place stress on you, the caregiver, making burnout a real possibility. Another real possibility is that someone will lose their temper to such an extent that they take it out on your loved one, maybe even physically. Not everyone can fully understand that they cannot help it.

You will often find yourself in the middle of the conflict, trying to keep peace and trying to do the best for your loved one. You will be trying to do the job of carer as well as spouse and/or parent. Your well-being will be severely taxed and you face a real prospect of a mental or physical breakdown.

It will be better for everyone, at this stage, to place the loved one in a care facility. The family unit will gather peace around themselves and your loved one will get the care that they deserve without upsetting everyone else. As the disease progresses, behavioral problems will increase, causing more stress on the caregiver.

If the patient is moved to a care facility, it will release some of the caregiver's pressure but other pressures will occur. You are still an important cog in the care wheel.

- When booking them into the care facility you have chosen, let the staff know of any food preferences or needs, like vegetarianism or gluten intolerance, and so on. They will also need their medical background and their medication. At last, you will be able to rest easily as their medications will be taken care of.
- You need to visit regularly. After all, you have a lot of freed-up time now that they are no longer at home.

If the care facility is close by, you can visit on a daily basis. You need to be able to let the family know that they are being well looked after and you can't do that if you do not do a regular check-up. Vary the time of your visit so that the staff is aware that you could pop in at any time. You could even settle them in for the night. There have been horrific posts of loved ones being mistreated and you want to make sure that they are getting the care that they deserve, no matter how many patients require attention or how impossible their behavior could be at any time. The staff needs to know that you are vigilant. Fortunately, most staff are very well-screened to ensure that they will be empathetic carers.

- Examine and question any bruises you may see. They will have probably forgotten the circumstances that gave them the bruise but it is well that the staff know you are observant. It is also possible that they may be a victim of other patients. Be aware of any difference in the way they behave. They may flinch when a specific person comes near but be fine with others. Question the staff as to why that is.

- If you hold the power of attorney, then you will have to manage everything for your loved one as well as take care of your own affairs. But you were probably doing that already.

- Be prepared for tirades when you visit them. They could accuse you of not caring for them anymore and that's why you abandoned them. You can't give in to these demands to be taken home and you must not feel that you have failed them. While the change for them is new, they will cry and ask to be taken home. The likelihood is that if you do bring them home, they will not recognize it and will berate you for tricking them. Just remember that you have chosen something that is good for the entire family. I know it is hard but you have to be strong.

- Be aware that there will be people, maybe in your own family, who will chastise you for "giving up" on your relative. And you will also face comments like, "Well, I took care of my mother until she passed. She did so much for me, so it was time for me to pay back." Do not let it stress you, obliterate them and their comments. You have been wonderful coping up to now. You have definitely earned your angel wings.

RESIDENTIAL CARE FACILITIES

There are four different types of facilities.

Assisted Living

This type of facility is only suitable if the patient is capable of living alone and fending for themself to a certain extent. It offers room and board, so they do not have to worry about cooking for themselves. There is a certain amount of supportive care. It bridges the gap between living at home and a nursing home. There is too much freedom for a stage 6 patient. It is a suitable solution for stages 1 through 5.

Nursing Homes

These places are sometimes referred to as skilled nursing care homes, long-term care homes, or custodial care homes. The patient has round-the-clock care should they need it. There is a medical staff to take care of medical problems and a therapy department to take care of bodily aches as well as mental stimulation. This type of care facility is suitable for stages 5 onwards.

Memory Care Units

These units are also known as special care units. They could be a part of a nursing home or they could be a stand-alone facility. They offer specialized, highly supervised care for dementia patients. The staff is equipped to handle medical needs as well as behavioral needs. They also have a fully functional therapy department.

Continuing Care Retirement Communities

These communities offer amenities that extend from inde-pendent living to frail care units where your loved one can receive all the care needed for the end stages of dementia. All kinds of medical care are available. If the move is made in the early stages, the patient will acclimate effortlessly to the new home. When the time comes to move into the frail care area, it will be easier because they will still be in familiar territory.

SELECTING A RESIDENTIAL CARE FACILITY

Selecting the right place for your loved one could be time-consuming, but you will be happy when you know that you have done your homework before choosing the final destination for your loved one.

You will first need to do research to find out what facilities are close to you. You do not want to get a facility that is too far away for regular visits. Chat with people who may have experience with these to help you to narrow down the possibilities. Once you have the names of a few places, go online and look at reviews for them.

When you have your list, make an appointment to visit them. It will be a good idea if you get another person to go with you to have more vision of the choice. Once the appointment is set, prepare a list of questions to ask. The Alzheimer's Association has excellent guidelines with a list of questions and things to look for when you visit the facility. These include questions on:

- Family involvement and communication: How involved can we be?

- Staffing expertise and amount of medical care provided: How well are the medical staff equipped to handle dementia patients?
- Are additional programs or services available? What activities are in place to keep the patient occupied during the day (Alzheimer's Association, 2023a)?

Be sure to find out the monthly cost plus any additional costs that may occur. You will be aware that you need to take care of the patient's hygienic needs and clothing but question if there is anything else you need to provide.

Residential care facilities should be part of a rating system regarding the quality and level of care that the patients receive. Your local health department or council should have this information. The Medicare website has information on nursing homes in your area.

Most facilities have a waiting list as dementia care units are in short supply. Get your loved one's name on the list as soon as possible; do not wait for the issue to become critical.

COST OF RESIDENTIAL CARE

You will be paying for the room, three meals a day, something to eat and drink at 10 and then again at 4 o'clock, and possibly something before bed. You will also be paying for medical care, giving medication, and various forms of therapy on an almost daily basis. So yes, it will be expensive. In 2021 an estimated figure was $7,000 per month for a memory care facility and $10,000 for a private room in a nursing home. But when you consider that $25 per hour will pay for a carer, the above costs are not that steep. Steep or not, it is still left to the family to foot the bills as your Medicare insurance will not cover it. Medicaid will only pay for long-term care for the impoverished, so most people are left to find their own solutions. Money will have to be found or maybe pooled from all family members. The patient hopefully had a 401k while they were working and this resource can be tapped. Other options are:

- Cash in any assets that the patient may have. These could be the family home, any properties, or other investments owned by the patient.
- Cash in any savings that the patient might have.
- Get the family to pool their resources.
- Check your loved one's insurance policies to see if one of them could be used to help support them.
- If they served in the military, you could see if the Veterans Association could help out.

If all of the above still does not give you enough funds, you could try Medicaid, which has restricted requirement policies. They will supply a list of facilities that they are prepared to subsidize. You might already have crossed these off for being unsuitable in some aspect; for instance, it might be an inconvenient distance from home.

PITFALLS AND PRECAUTIONS

Your loved one has lost all sense of staying safe. They are curious about things lying around as they feel they have never seen this new implement before. They will not know how to operate it and will be totally oblivious to any danger that may come with it being used. In this, they are very much like a child.

- Some hazardous products look so good. Just think of the beautiful color that defines Methylated spirits. They may think it is a delicious drink. So childproofing the house becomes normal again. All poisonous substances must be kept under lock and key.
- Dangerous or potential weapons must also be kept under lock and key. If there is a gun in the home, keep the bullets and the gun in different places but still keep the gun in a safe, secure place.
- There is a high risk that the patient will fall as their balance and movement is bad. A walking stick or a walker is the solution for support when you cannot hang onto them.
- Their eyesight will also be failing, making it difficult to get around. They will get bruises from bumping into tables, doors, and other furniture.
- Their confusion will lead to disorientation which will upset them.

- Their movements will be compromised as their coordination is declining.

WHAT SHOULD WE PREPARE FOR NEXT?

As your loved one drifts into the next and final stage, there will be rapid degradation of all bodily functions, and 24-hour care is essential. The patient will probably be bound to his bed. Their understanding and logical thought will rapidly disappear.

6

STAGE 7 (SEVERE DEMENTIA)

This is the final stage for your loved one. Care must be 24/7, so if you have not yet organized full-time care for your loved one, it must be done now. The strain and pressure that you felt before will be more than doubled if you try to do this yourself. The end of life is close and you have done all in your power for your loved one. You now need to spend a bit more time on self-care while a nurse or carer takes over the harder duties. The care takes on another aspect—the need to keep the patient comfortable, warm, and fed. The focus is on end-of-life care. It is hard and heartbreaking to watch the degradation and helplessness of that once-strong person.

CHARACTERISTICS OF STAGE 7

This final heart-breaking stage sees the degradation of all normal activity. Their ability to talk, listen, and think is severely impacted. There is also a decline in what the patient is able to achieve physically.

CHANGES IN YOUR LOVED ONE

The changes that were observed before have now escalated to the extent that your loved one loses the ability to

- respond to their environment.
- distinguish between hot and cold weather.
- eat, speak, and swallow.
- carry on a viable conversation.
- control movement.
- change from seated to standing and back.
- point out where they have pain.
- go to the toilet without help.
- recognize when they need the toilet.

You could observe extreme personality changes. So apart from them probably not recognizing you, you will find it hard to find a vestige of your loved one's personality. Here are some of the personality changes that may happen:

- They may be easily upset, which could turn into anger quite quickly.
- They may start hallucinating. The things they see may frighten or amuse them.
- They may indulge in restless pacing around the room.
- They will be quick to accuse people of stealing when they can't find something. They will have forgotten that they put it in a safe place.
- They may resort to physical violence. This will probably be due to their inability to express themselves with words.
- They could become depressed, even if this was not something they had experienced before (NIH, 2017).

Your loved one, at this stage, will need help with everything from eating, going to the toilet, and taking medications. As the muscles in their body deteriorate, you will find that they battle to

- walk
- talk
- swallow food and medications

They become more frail. Their body's immunity will decrease. No one should visit if they have a cold or flu. If they catch what's going around, it could quickly change to pneumonia, and with their lack of immunity, it could be a serious condition. They are going to need round-the-clock care. Serious medical conditions could appear suddenly.

Your communication with them will have to be adjusted. Words are becoming incomprehensible, so you need to find other means of soothing them. You could play music. If you play music from when they were a teen or a tune that they enjoyed and have memories of, they may well respond to it. If you want to soothe them out of a mood, play soft, relaxing music. They may also respond to a gentle touch.

If they need more care than you or the home can give them, it might be time to consider Hospice. They have experience dealing with end-of-life matters and will be a support for you and the other family members when the time comes to say a final goodbye.

YOUR CHANGING ROLE

Because your loved one is no longer capable of verbalizing their needs, you need to be vigilant to help them when they need help. You are going to rely on what you can observe in them. You will find that your intuition kicks in, allowing you to intuitively anticipate their needs. Don't delay calling in medical expertise if the situation calls for it.

There is nothing you can do to change the progression of the disease but you can keep them calm and pain-free. They may be spending a large portion of the day in bed or in a wheel-chair, so bedsores become a definite possibility. In order to prevent bed sores from forming, help your loved one to change position to minimize friction on one part of the body. Keep their skin dry and moisturized. You will need to examine their skin on a daily basis. Bedsores can form on the bony areas of the skin. Untreated bed sores can cause a severe infection that your loved one's body cannot handle.

Some days you may not get any response from them. If this happens, remain calm and talk soothingly. They may be able to hear you and your calmness and it may run off onto them.

Earlier in the disease, you hopefully addressed end-of-life choices. You need to revisit them now as there may be changes due to the progress of the disease. If you decide to move your loved one to a hospice, these documents will be needed. The staff there will help you fill in any blanks you may have missed when you generated the documents. They will request that you have a DNR in place should the patient deteriorate. Make sure you also have a few copies you can give to concerned family members and the patient's doctors, and remember to keep one for yourself.

Caring for your loved one gives you a sense of purpose in this difficult time. As you go about the day, you will add new skills to your repertoire while adding more purpose to the loved one's life. Your support helps the loved one adjust to the new norms of his life.

As they pass through the various stages, they may need to be reminded who you are. When in a conversation with them, talk slowly and listen carefully. If they question why a deceased family member isn't coming to visit, tell them a white lie, "She's not here right now" rather than the truth, "She died ten years ago." You may have to repeat things numerous times as they will forget things quickly. Keep your cool; they are able to recognize body language, so be careful of showing impatience, annoyance, or any other bad reaction to what they are saying, even though they have said the same thing numerous times.

Don't try to prompt their memory by saying something like "Don't you remember?" or "I just told you."

When there are visitors, don't ignore your loved one by focusing all your attention on the visitor. Include them in the visit by addressing remarks to them as well as to the visitor. And never discuss their disease as if they aren't there— they will hear everything and be hurt that they are being ignored.

Taking Care of Yourself

Keeping yourself healthy has always been a priority but it is more so now. If you fall sick, your loved one will have to get used to a new carer which is going to be difficult for them. Remember that you are important to your loved one; you give them stability in their unstable world.

Challenges

Caring for your loved one takes time away from the other loves in your life as well as your job. The rest of your family may get resentful of the time you spend with your loved one. You are so focussed on your loved one that you stand in peril of burnout. You must find time for the other family members and, more importantly, yourself.

If you gave up your job to be a caregiver, you may be resentful. You must make sure that your charge does not pick up on your frustrations. You might also be worried about finances since giving up your job. You might also be worried about getting your job (or a similar one) back.

The one thing you crave is to have the help and support of your close family members.

IS HOSPICE RIGHT FOR ME, MY FAMILY AND MY LOVED ONE?

You have two choices for Stage 7 nursing—Hospice and palliative care.

Palliative Care

Palliative care helps the patient and their family deal with a life-threatening illness. It encompasses spiritual, psychological, physical, and social needs. The primary caregiver will be relieved of most of their duties.

When the patient enters palliative care, they have a wealth of professionals available to them. This team of professionals will take over the medical care, giving the caregiver time to devote to sharing these last months with their loved one.

Palliative care will usually be given in a hospital setting because a hospital has all the facilities and equipment that may be needed. The bills will have to be paid by the family unless the patient has private insurance that will cover the costs.

Hospice

Hospice gives end-of-life care. Admission into a hospice usually occurs when a doctor has given a patient up to six more months of life. You can often apply to Medicare or Medicaid to help with the bills but it would help financially if the patient had private insurance.

Hospice staff can help the patient in many settings. If you choose to keep the patient at home, they will do home visits. They will also care for the patient in a hospital, nursing home, or in their own Hospice houses.

Hospice care includes respite care for the caregiver. The staff can organize chaplain visits and grief counseling. The staff are trained to help all family members accept the situation before the death of their loved one and they are also there to help after death.

Most families who used a hospice in the final stages of the disease have said that they should have utilized a hospice earlier.

PITFALLS OF STAGE 7

Health conditions that plagued the patient in the past could easily recur. Their body is no longer capable of fighting infections; a cold could quickly turn into bronchitis or pneumonia. It is doubtful that they could make a full recovery. Other conditions like hypertension could get worse.

Falls, cuts, and bruises will appear suddenly and as suddenly spiral out of control. As the body's immune system is compromised, it is doubtful that the patient will survive these injuries, even if they appear minor.

Bed sores could become infected if not treated timeously.

If your loved one is agitated, they may be in pain, and unfortunately, they are not able to tell you what is wrong. You need to do a full body check as well as a check on their surroundings. Don't be alarmed if they try to fight you off, as they don't know who is family and who is a stranger.

Encourage them to drink water, tea, or coffee, as dehydration is a real concern. As they are drinking, check that they are swallowing the beverage, as their swallowing reflex no longer works so well.

PREPARING FOR END OF LIFE

The general estimation of Stage 7 is between one and two years. Let the family and close friends know that their loved one has entered Stage 7 of the disease and end of life is imminent. You will need to warn them again that their loved one will not know who they are but may think they are his mother, father, spouse, or other relative. They will also have lost memory of places they have been to or lived in. They will have no memory of events. Invite them to come and say their goodbyes but don't be upset if they refuse the invite. Not everyone is as strong as you. Many would rather remember them for who they were rather than see them as they are now.

Coach those who will put in an appearance. Too many visitors at a time will confuse your loved one and they may get angry with all these strangers in their room. Allow only two to three extra people in the room. Try to limit the number of visits per day. Ask them to keep their visit light natured. Tell them to talk a bit slower than normal to give your loved one time to process what is being said. Remind them to keep their sentences simple. If visitors have a cold or flu, suggest they come another time or wear a surgical mask in their room.

As the end of life approaches, you will find that your loved one sleeps most of the time. This is natural. Their energy sources are depleted and frequent naps will give them time to rebuild their energy. It is very likely that during a nap, they will drift off, away from the pain, the confusion, and the helplessness.

During these last days, don't forget to take care of yourself. You and the other close family members need grief counseling to help you face the inevitable when it happens. The grief counselor will help you over the days following the death of the patient. Although death is part of life and normally, people will not seek counseling, the grief that you and your family have had to contend with has built up over the years that dementia settled in your loved one. Remember that hospice will be able to help you handle this period of time.

SIGNS THAT END OF LIFE IS NEAR

Although there will be gradual indications throughout Stage 7, when the end of life is a few days away, you can prepare yourself by observing the changes in your loved one. Changes could be:

- They are not interested in food or drink. However, you must keep them hydrated. This could be difficult as they may have trouble swallowing. Moistening their lips or allowing them to suck on some ice chips will help get some liquid into their system. Do not try to force-feed them. Food is not important at this time.
- They will be very weak and will not be able to move from their bed. They will need help with everything.

- They may become disorientated. They may find it hard to follow what you or visitors are saying. They may drift in and out of consciousness. Alternatively, they may become restless. This restlessness is called "terminal restlessness" (Social Care Institute for Excellence, 2020).

As the disease takes over, Their breathing will become labored and irregular. Every now and then, their breathing may stop for a few seconds before starting up again. Their feet and hands will be cold and may turn blue as the flow of blood around the body deteriorates. These signs that you can observe are distressing for the family but your loved one is not aware of the symptoms (Alzheimer's Society, 2019).

At this stage, all you can do is to ensure that your loved one is comfortable and not in any pain as the body shuts down, releasing both of you.

The symptoms discussed above could be a sign of the end of life or it could be due to an infection. It is best to ask for a medical opinion, as your loved one could have a treatable condition. A medical professional will be aware of the patient's DNR wishes. But if the patient's condition is a result of an infection, the doctor will treat the infection.

PROFESSIONAL HELP FOR END OF LIFE

Healthcare professionals can be your anchor in the storm that is happening around you. They can help you come to terms with the limited time available to you. Their main job will, of course, be the patient, but you will also benefit from their care. You can take rest breaks while they see to your loved one.

They can treat your loved one's pain, restlessness, and distress. They have the authority to medicate. If your loved one is having difficulty swallowing, the medication can be given intravenously. They could also use injections or a skin patch. Medication can also be provided via a syringe pump which has a small needle under the skin.

Earlier in the disease, you would have made sure that your loved one had given you instructions about their end-of-life preferences. If they named people they would like to see for the last time, you need to make sure that they are there for your loved one. If they were religious, call for their priest, minister, rabbi, or other spiritual leader.

7

AFTERWARDS—MOVING TOWARD RECOVERY

The last few years have now come to an end. Your job as a caregiver is over. The final weeks of your loved one's life were fairly hectic. Now suddenly, you have lost the job that kept you busy and on your toes for so long. You will grieve over the loss of your loved one but there will also be a sense of loss over the job that is now over. At first, you will feel lost and you will wonder how you will fill the days. But this won't last long as there will be a lot of things that have to be dealt with. But before you start on that, you need to devote some time to healing yourself. Take a day or two to pamper yourself in any way that appeals to you.

WHAT HAPPENS NOW?

The estate will be settled by the person who was nominated as executor. This could take a few months or a few years, depending on the complexity of it. You may have been made the executor. If someone else has been named as the executor, you may have to work with them. Anyone could be named as the executor, even if that person is also a beneficiary of the will. If you are named executor, you can refuse it if you so choose. The executor's duties are to ensure that the deceased's wishes, as stated in his will, are followed to the letter.

It is always preferable to go through an attorney as they deal with many cases like this. The deceased might have housed his will with a legal firm, in which case, you have all the help you need. If you do not have an attorney, you could apply to your local Clerk of the Court to help you through the maze of things that need to be done. There are many things that you can deal with without legal counsel:

1. Find the will. This could be easy if you had that conversation with your loved one. However, they could have changed the place as dementia patients often hide things and forget where they have hidden it. You may have to search for it in drawers, a safe, or a safety depository box. If your loved one had a lawyer, it might be in their office. Hopefully, they would have made a will; if not, they died intestate. If this is the case, you will need legal help.

2. You will need to file the will with your local probate court. Before filing it with the court, make sure you have a copy.

3. Notify all businesses that your loved one had accounts with. This is necessary as they need to be aware that outstanding payments will be dealt with by the estate. Notify

- banks to stop automatic payments.
- utility departments to suspend the account.
- credit card companies.
- clothing stores.
- the cable company.
- the internet service provider.
- any other place that the deceased had dealings with.

Just be aware that if the deceased's spouse is still alive, she may need access to the above.

4. Make an inventory of all the contents of the home. This is to help when you come to split the items with the beneficiaries. You will need an appraiser to help you evaluate all the items.

5. A lawyer will help you through this step. You may need to get probate which is a legal document allowing the executor to divide up the estate in accordance with the will of the deceased. A lawyer will guide you as to whether you need probate or not. If the deceased left both a will and a living trust, you will need to work with the appointed trustee. A

living trust does not need probate before the beneficiaries are given the properties.

6. Let the other beneficiaries be aware of what is happening with the estate. If they feel you are incompetent, they could go to a court of law to have you removed as executor. This will only happen if you are not upfront with what is happening to the will.

7. Ensure that the deceased's assets are safe. If it is a house, make sure that the gardens are looked after. Jewelry must be placed in a safe place, as will any other valuable possessions.

8. Collect any money that is due to the estate. It would be a good idea to open a bank account in the estate's name.

9. Settle any outstanding amounts or ask the companies to wait until the state is wound up. If there is no ready money in the estate, you do not have to dig deep in your own pocket to settle the bills. You may need to get a lawyer to act for you or take it to court to help you figure out which bills take priority.

10. Check up on unpaid taxes. Fill in a tax return for the deceased. You may also have to pay property tax.

11. When all the above has been taken care of, you can split the estate according to the will.

12. The estate can now be finalized and closed. You will need to prepare a final accounting of the estate. This includes all financial transactions mentioned above. When this is

complete, a copy must be lodged with the probate court. Each beneficiary will also receive a copy, and you need to retain a copy for yourself.

Animals

Animals form a large part of our lives. If the deceased had animals, you need to make a decision about them if they have not been included in the will. An animal will also be grieving. Suddenly their whole routine has changed. Strange people are wafting around and their owner is nowhere to be found. They will be bewildered. I saw a video of a cat nuzzling a cell phone that was playing a video of her deceased owner. The love that the cat had for the owner was touching. This could have been one of the issues you encouraged your loved one to settle. In a will, there should be a space for what you want to happen to your pets.

If the estate is a farm or a small holding, the animals there need to be looked after while the estate is pending. Again there could have been provisions for the animals in the will. The family is grieving and may not even remember to care for the animals but hopefully, one of the mourners will remember and take on the job of caring for the animals. The person who has been caring for the animals up to now may be interested in taking them on.

Medications

When clearing up, you will come across his supply of medicines. There may be some, like painkillers, that you can use but the medications that were for his disease need to be disposed of. You can't flush them down the toilets as that water eventually finds its way into rivers or seas, killing anything that is trying to survive. So what options are available to you? Many pharmacists will take them back for free disposal to patients who cannot afford medicine. If they do not repurpose them, they will probably be able to give them to a medical disposal company. You could ask your doctor for further advice.

Personal Items

Some of these items will not have been used for a while but they could still have sensitive information on them. So round up any computer equipment your loved one had, desktop, laptop, or tablet. They probably also had a cell phone.

Their banking details will probably be on the computer. These must be deleted as soon as possible with permission from the executor.

The computer will also help you find any services that need to be canceled, like Netflix, Zoom, and personal email accounts.

Spreading the News

The caregiver at this stage may be feeling tired. There is so much still to do. So now is the time for the family to rally around. Again it would have been better to sort this out before the event but now is as good a time as any. Nominate someone to take care of informing everyone. That person could delegate a few family members with the task of personally contacting family and friends. Acquaintances could be informed via a newspaper in the obituary column. Split the task with members of the family. Make sure that all people who were close to the deceased are contacted. Your loved one's cell phone will help establish this.

As you spread the news via newspapers, be aware that criminals keep a beady eye on the obituary column. They pick up names and addresses and look out for when the funeral takes place. They hope that the home is left unattended while everyone is at the funeral service. You need to get a volunteer to stay in the house so it is occupied and hopefully will deter the thief from attempting a housebreaking. It's a great little task to give to someone who asks, "What can I do to help?" but doesn't really have the capacity to be very physically involved.

GRIEVE

Some people may say that the correct time to grieve is one year, others may say five years, but I say that grief has no time limit. The amount of time needed to grieve is very personal. What works for one person may not work for another. Most firms will only give up to three days' leave which is crazy.

Now, at the end of this part of your journey, you have:

- lost a loved one
- lost your job as a caregiver
- lost your identity

Your job as a caregiver kept you busy for most of the day and sometimes well into the night. Now you suddenly have all this free time that you don't know how to fill. For so many years, you have been a helper, and it has almost robbed you of your identity, so you need to find what it is that makes you tick.

As you grieve, you may experience feelings of emptiness. Your sleep cycle may be disrupted and you may lose your appetite. You could alternate your feelings from deep sadness to anger. There is no right way to grieve. You may find that you grieve anew at birthdays, certain aromas, or events.

As you go through the process, you will pass through the following stages:

1. Denial that the person is no longer there
2. Anger at the deceased, the world, and maybe your supreme being
3. Bargaining with a deity
4. Depression, and finally
5. Acceptance (Cox, 2022)

Here are some coping tips while you are still in the first stage:

- Join a support group.
- Crying will help you get rid of the feelings jammed up inside you.
- Ask friends or family to help you.
- Don't try to do everything at once—prioritize.
- Write about it.
- Follow a passion (Fletcher, 2023).

Give yourself permission to grieve and concentrate on memories of your loved one before dementia entered his life.

POST-TRAUMATIC CAREGIVER STRESS DISORDER (PCSD)

When you were caring for your loved one, it seemed to engulf your whole life. When they died, you suddenly had too much time. You may feel anxious and lost. Some people have reported that they suddenly developed panic attacks and most acknowledge sinking into depression.

Your grief actually started quite a long time ago. Death has just given you permission to grieve openly.

You had to deal with stress during your time as a caregiver, which affected you emotionally, physically, and spiritually. While caring for your loved one, you probably often felt that the situation was hopeless and that you couldn't do anything to reverse the disease made you feel helpless. And all the time you are watching the patient deteriorate, you are dealing with grief for the person they once were.

You need to acknowledge your feelings, even those that make you uncomfortable. Many caregivers experience a feeling of relief. And as can be expected, they will feel guilty for having those feelings. It may be an idea to get some grief counseling. With grief counseling, you will understand that relief is a perfectly normal response. A good place to get that counseling is with hospice-trained staff. You may feel that you could have done more for your loved one and you can't forgive yourself. No matter how ideal a caregiver you have been, I've yet to meet a survivor that didn't feel they should have done more. Caregiver grief is an oddly twisted emotional rollercoaster!

The trained staff will help you see that you did everything that was humanly possible for your loved one.

Everything that you are feeling is perfectly normal. The trauma symptoms will go away when you understand why you have those feelings.

Sharing your feelings in a support group will help you come to terms with the situation. If you are able, consider writing it all down to share with others who are in the same situation.

And above all, take care of yourself physically, mentally, and spiritually. Recovery may take years, but you are worth it. You need to realize that everything you did was enough; you could not have done more. It is normal to feel a sense of loneliness. It comes from the suddenness that you lost your position as a caregiver. You need to find something to fill that void. Pick up with friends you may have neglected in the past few years. If they are true friends, they will welcome you back with open arms.

The next chapter of your life is about you! Spoil yourself; join an exercise class. Meet new people. Catch up on the years of lost sleep.

YOUR CHANCE TO HELP ANOTHER CAREGIVER

I wish you didn't know how hard this journey is… But I know you do, and that means you're in a unique position to help someone else.

Simply by sharing your honest opinion of this book and a little about your own experience as a caregiver, you'll show new readers where they can find the support they're looking for.

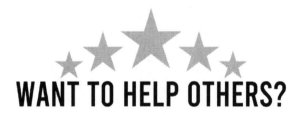

Thank you so much for your help. Remember: You're doing an amazing job, and you should be proud. Your loved one would be.

Scan the QR code to leave a review on Amazon!

CONCLUSION

I hope you are better equipped now than you were before we started this trip together. I don't know which form of dementia your loved one has or had but the explanations in chapter 1 went over the main dementia diseases. Although the various diseases cause damage in different areas of the brain, the end result is generally the same.

Each of the seven stages of dementia has been discussed in detail, giving you facts to grab onto while nursing your loved one.

- Stages 1–3 are probably not even diagnosed. You, being close to your loved one, will notice small changes in them, which are not enough to cause concern. When they forget someone or something, that can be put down to the normal aging process but you maybe had an inkling that this was a bit more serious. By the time they were reaching the end of Stage 3, you will have realized that there is more to their problem than normal aging.

- When they reach Stage 4, the disease is able to be identified as dementia, and an MRI or other brain scan will point the medical advisor in the right direction. Stage 4 sees forgetfulness increasing. It might even go as far as forgetting the names of certain family members.

- Stage 5 brings in disorientation and confusion as well as more memory loss. While long-term memory is still active, your loved one will forget things that happened a few days ago. They will forget his address and phone number. Wandering may occur. This is problematic as they will forget how to get home and be unable to tell anyone where they live. So you will need to tighten the reins.

- The dementia has gained strength in Stage 6. Short-term memory has gone and long-term memory becomes sketchy. Wandering becomes a real threat and sleeping cycles will be disrupted. They now need full-time attendance.

- Stage 7 is the final stage. They will need help with everything. They battle to swallow, so feeding must either be purees like baby food or intravenous feeding.

All through this, you have been the principal caregiver. I've said it before but it needs to be repeated: you are important to them, so you must look after yourself. Nap when they nap and get a night nurse so that you can get a good night's sleep. Your loved one needs to have everything done for them, so a day nurse is a definite option for you.

A hospice is your go-to place for advice and care in the form of visiting nurses or a bed in a hospice home. When your loved one has passed away, the hospice will help you in your grief.

At the end, look back on what you did for your loved one, which is a lot. Do not look back and try to see what you could have done better. You did the best that you could. Hold your head up proudly. You will have many different emotions. One might be a relief for you and for the recently deceased. You both have been through a tough time for many years, so don't berate yourself for feeling relief. It might take time for you to recenter yourself within the family again.

I hope my experiences and the information in this book have been cathartic for you. If you feel so inclined and the book has helped you, could you leave a review, please?

ADDITIONAL RESOURCES

As our understanding of dementia grows, so does the amount of information available to those living with the disease, their caregivers, family, and friends. Here are a few resources to explore further.

ORGANIZATIONS

Government-sponsored Research and Information in the US

- Centers for Disease Control and Prevention (CDC) —The CDC's Alzheimer's Disease and Healthy Aging program provides information on a range of topics related to dementia and cognitive health in the US senior population. This site is primarily concerned with Alzheimer's disease, as it is the most common dementia. However, almost everything they report is applicable to all types of dementia.

- NIH National Institute on Aging (NIA)—A division of the National Institute of Health, NIA is a source of information on a variety of issues impacting the senior population, including dementia. It provides information on Alzheimer's Disease Research Centers (ADRC) throughout the US.

Medical and Research Centers in the US

There are numerous centers around the US with groundbreaking research and supportive treatment programs. These are considered among the tops in the field.

- Johns Hopkins Hospital (Baltimore, MD). Once you have entered the website, you will see a search option on the top right-hand side. Type in dementia and select one of the eight sections.
- Mount Sinai Medical Center (New York, NY). The search button gives you access to 10 sections on dementia.
- Ronald Reagan UCLA Medical Center (Los Angeles, CA). There is a wealth of information on dementia. The quickest way to get your options is to do a search.
- Cleveland Clinic/Aging Brain Clinic (Cleveland, OH). This clinic specializes in treating the affected

patient as well as giving support and understanding to family and close friends.

- Massachusetts General Hospital/Geriatrics Unit (Boston, MA) offers collaborative care to the patient and the family.
- Mayo Clinic (Rochester, MN). To read the information on Dementia, select "D" from the displayed alphabet and then scroll until you find "dementia."
- Duke University Medical Center (Durham, NC). Once you search for dementia, you will get many hyperlinks taking you to a specific section of dementia. An interesting section is their bereavement options.
- NYU Langone Medical Center (New York, NY). This site has reports of clinical trials and other titbits of information once you have searched for dementia.
- University of Pittsburgh Medical Center/Alzheimer's Disease Research Center (ADRC) (Pittsburgh, PA). You can find reports of their research in this area.

Support, Research Funding, and Information

- Alzheimer's Association. This website deals with specific caregiver advice. The stages of Alzheimer's are discussed. If your loved one has one of the other types of dementia, it will follow similar lines. The website will also guide you to support groups in your area.

- Alzheimer's Drug Discovery Foundation. If you are looking for facts and figures as well as descriptions of the disease, this is the site for you.
- Alzheimer's Foundation of America. This site offers help to caregivers as well as the sufferer. They run on donations, so the site includes a link to help you donate. They have staff on call 24/7.
- The American Brain Foundation deals with all types of brain malfunctions. They hold events, publish papers, and are heavily involved in trying to find a cure. They believe that all brain diseases share common issues and if they find the key to one brain disease, it will help all.
- Bright Focus is involved in research on many types of afflictions, including brain diseases.
- Cure Alzheimer's Fund. This non-profit organization funds research on Alzheimer's disease. They are looking at ways to either prevent it or slow down its progress. They are also looking at the possibility of reversing the damage.
- The Dementia Society of America looks at all aspects of dementia and offers help and guidance, and brings hope to caregivers. They have a month;y newspaper that will keep you up to date on recent research.

- Dementia Spring Foundation explores the use of the arts in treating dementia. There are articles specifically for caregivers.
- Hospice Foundation of America offers support for the patient and the carer. Their focus is on giving a good quality of life in the end stages.
- Lewy Body Dementia Association has a mission to help the families and caregivers of patients who have Lewy Body Dementia. If you sign up on the website, you will be kept updated on the current research.

BOOKS

Many of these books are available in a variety of formats, including hardback, paperback, e-book, and audiobook. A few have been translated into Spanish. As of this writing, all are in print and available on Amazon.

General Information

- *The 36-Hour Day: A Family Guide to Caring for People Who Have Alzheimer's Disease, Related Dementias* (7th Edition, 2021) by Nancy L. Mace & Peter V. Rabins —Although this book was first published over 40 years ago, this updated edition remains the gold standard for information on all phases of dementia. It recognizes the challenges that you, the patient, and the family will be going through. It also looks at the financial and legal side of things. This reference book is highly recommended by many caregivers, supportive organizations, and healthcare professionals.

- *Activities to do with Your Parent Who has Alzheimer's Dementia* (2014) by Judith A. Levy—This user-friendly book has practical activities that help preserve the patient's skills in self-care, mobility, and socialization. When one is caring for a dementia patient, you are sometimes hard-pressed to find enough to do that is within his capabilities. With this book, you no longer have to stress.

- *The Best Friends Approach to Dementia Care* (2016) by Virginia Bell and David Troxel—Focuses on a relationship-centered approach to dementia care—one that emphasizes respect, support, empathy, and trust. It also has a chapter on activities. It is a good resource for caregivers and family members of dementia patients.

- *Creating Moments of Joy Along the Alzheimer's Journey: A Guide for Families and Caregivers* (5th Edition, 2016) by Jolene Brackey—Another beloved bestseller that has been expanded and updated. The author's vision of creating small moments of joy even in the midst of difficult days mixes practical advice with a dose of encouragement and humor. A dementia patient will forget what you did or said, but the feeling they had at that time will remain with them. It is written from the patient's perspective.

- *The Dementia Handbook: How to Provide Dementia Care at Home* (2017) by Judy Cornish—The author is the creator of the DAWN Method; the straightforward language gives families an understanding of the cognitive changes and shifting abilities that shape the patient's reality. The book gives a roadmap to both the carer and the patient. It is also available in Spanish!

- *Learning to Speak Alzheimer's: A Groundbreaking Approach for Everyone Dealing with the Disease* (2004) by Joanne Koenig-Coste and Robert N. Butler, M.D. —The book has a practical approach that emphasizes relating to patients in their reality; her proven method enhances communication between caregiver and patients. The book gives many tips on how to deal with specific issues. The author talks from a deep experience.

- *Managing Alzheimer's and Dementia Behaviors: Common Sense Caregiving* (2012) by Gary Joseph LeBlanc —Whether you are a healthcare professional or a family caregiver, this book expands our understanding of what the patient is going through and fosters better communication. It is an easy read while giving many tips along the way.

- *Thoughtful Dementia Care: Understanding the Dementia Experience* (2012) by Jennifer Ghent-Fuller—An easy-to-read portrayal of the world of dementia with insights and practical suggestions for those living on the frontlines of caregiving for a loved one. Some of the topics are explained from the patient's point of view, which is rather unique.

Health and Nutrition

- *The Alzheimer's Action Plan: What You Need to Know—and What You Can Do—About Memory Problems, from Prevention to Early Intervention and Care* (2009) by P. Murali Doraiswamy, M.D., Lisa P. Gwyther, M.S.W., and Tina Adler—Through the combined insights of a world-class physician and an award-winning social worker, readers gain valuable information on testing, clinical trials and understanding the future of Alzheimer's treatment. The subject is dealt with compassionately and with a touch of humor.
- *Nutrition for Brain Health: Fighting Dementia (Part of Alzheimer's Roadmap)* (2020) by Laura Town and Karen Kassel Hoffman—Understand the importance of nutrition in the prevention of dementia for those at risk and slowing of decline for those in the early stages of the disease. It contains checklists to help you build up a healthy shopping list.

Inspirational

- *Chicken Soup for the Soul: Living with Alzheimer's & Other Dementias: 101 Stories of Caregiving, Coping, and*

Compassion (2014) by Amy Newmark and Angela Timashenka—Part of the beloved series of inspiration writings, 101 stories offer support, advice, and comfort for both those living with dementia and their caregivers. The many personal stories are helpful to carers and patients alike. It is always comforting to find that you are not alone in dealing with this awful disease.

- *Dementia: Living in the Memories of God* (2012) by John Swinton—A compassionate pastoral response to dementia and the indignities of memory loss and disorientation. It is a helpful and encouraging book for Christian readers.

PODCASTS

- From Johns Hopkins' Memory and Alzheimer's Treatment Center—A collection of recommended podcasts from one of the leading medical centers in the research and treatment of dementia. When you access the John Hopkins website, click the search icon on the top right of the screen and search for Podcasts.
- *Dementia Untangled*—From Banner Health, this podcast explores the disease through conversations with doctors, experts, and community advocates on a variety of topics to create a supportive care community. To listen to the podcasts, Google *Dementia Untangled Podcast.*

- *Caregiver Storyteller*—From CaringKind, highlights the poignant stories of caregivers as they navigate the reality of caring for a loved one with dementia. These podcasts can be accessed when you Google *Caregiver Storyteller Podcast.*

FILMS AND DOCUMENTARIES

Film portrayals of dementia are often criticized for not going far enough in their depictions, but they can still help us to understand the toll the disease takes on everyone and help to open up difficult conversations among families. These are considered among the best. Many are available on your favorite streaming service.

Documentaries

- *Alive Inside* (2014)—Centers on the power of music as a healing balm and medicine for the soul for those living with dementia. It is available on YouTube for free.
- *First Cousin Once Removed* (2012)—Considered one of the finest documentaries made on the challenges and debilitations of Alzheimer's Disease. Amazon has the movie.

Dramas

- *Age Old Friends* (1989)—Two elderly friends contend with the frailties of mind and body as they fight to retain their independence in a nursing home. Due to its age, this film may be difficult to locate, although Amazon seems to have the DVD.

- *Aurora Borealis* (2005)—The story of a young man struggling with his place in the world who takes a job as a handyman in an apartment building to be closer to his grandfather, played by Donald Sutherland, who has Alzheimer's. Amazon may have the movie.

- *Away From Her* (2006)—A husband copes with his wife's Alzheimer's as well as her growing attachment to another man residing in her nursing home. Amazon has copies.

- *The Father* (2020)—This psychological drama plays heavily on the ruptured sense of reality dementia patients suffer. It is based on a French play starring Anthony Hopkins and Olivia Colman. Amazon Prime has the movie.

- *Iris* (2001)—This is a biographical drama about novelist Iris Murdoch and her husband as they struggle through her deteriorating dementia. It stars Judi Dench and Jim Broadbent. It is available on Google Play to rent or buy.

- *The Leisure Seeker* (2017)—A runaway couple makes one last epic road trip before his Alzheimer's and her cancer catch up with them. It stars Helen Mirren and Donald Sutherland. It is available on YouTube.

- *Poetry* (2010)—A woman develops an interest in poetry as she deals with an irresponsible grandson and her own Alzheimer's disease—a South Korean-French film with subtitles. Amazon has copies.

- *The Savages* (2007)—Considered a black comedy-drama, this film brings two estranged siblings together to care for their equally estranged elderly father, who is slipping deeper into dementia. It stars Laura Linney and Philip Seymour Hoffman. It is available on YouTube.

- *A Song for Martin* (2001)—A successful composer and violinist find each other in midlife, only to have Alzheimer's destroy their happiness—taking dignity and memory with it—a Swedish film with subtitles. Amazon has copies.

- *Still Alice* (2014)—Based on a novel by the same name, a respected professor must come face-to-face with her early-onset Alzheimer's. It stars Julianne Moore. It is available on Google Play.

- *What They Had* (2018)—A family is in crisis as they struggle with competing ideas—can a mom be kept at home or must she be placed in a nursing home? It stars Hilary Swank. It is available on Amazon.

ADDITIONAL INFORMATION

Dawn

The Dementia & Alzheimer's Wellbeing Network (DAWN) website provides support, coaching, training, and information to caregivers and families. Their approach to strength-based dementia care focuses on "less stress, more companionship, better communication."

We know that dementia patients lose the ability to do many things but certain techniques will still be remembered. If you can tap into those techniques, there will be hours of pleasure as you explore what they can do rather than what their limitations are.

The DAWN Method of Dementia Care channel on YouTube has a small collection of informative videos.

Rosalynn Carter Institute for Caregivers

Rosalynn Carter Institute for Caregivers was founded by former first lady Rosalynn Carter. She feels that everyone will be on one side of caregiving in their lifetime. They may be caregivers or may need a caregiver.

It is a non-profit organization that has championed the cause of unpaid caregivers for over 35 years through training, coaching, and advocacy. Their programs support the health, resilience, and strength of those unpaid caregivers who provide care for loved ones that are dealing with issues of aging, illness, or disability. High on their list of initiatives is support for those caring for loved ones with dementia.

In 2023, the RCI announced that their much-beloved founder has dementia. Despite this, she continues to serve as an inspiration for the Institute and millions of caregivers worldwide.

Teepa Snow and PAC Team

Teepa Snow is a respected dementia care specialist. Her Positive Approach to Care (PAC) Team offers education, support, and information. Their mission statement identifies the Team's goal of "using our talents and abilities to develop awareness, knowledge, and skill with all people, that will transform what exists into a more positive dementia care culture" (Snow, 2019).

Teepa Snow's Positive Approach to Care channel on YouTube has numerous short videos on dementia care.

REFERENCES

AgeSpace. (n.d.). *Everything you need to know about power of attorney*. Age Space. Retrieved July 22, 2023, from https://www.agespace.org/legal/power-of-attorney

Alzheimer's Association. (2019a). *Medical tests for diagnosing Alzheimer's*. Alzheimer's Disease and Dementia. https://www.alz.org/alzheimers-dementia/diagnosis/medical_tests

Alzheimer's Association. (2019b). *Types of dementia*. Alzheimer's Disease and Dementia. https://www.alz.org/alzheimers-dementia/what-is-dementia/types-of-dementia

Alzheimer's Association. (2022). *What is Alzheimer's? Alzheimer's Disease and Dementia*. Alzheimer's Association. https://www.alz.org/alzheimers-dementia/what-is-alzheimers

Alzheimer's Association. (2023a). *Alzheimer's disease facts and figures*. Alzheimer's Association. https://www.alz.org/media/Documents/alzheimers-facts-and-figures.pdf

Alzheimer's Association. (2023b, April). *Choosing a residential care community*. https://Alz.org/Media/Documents/Alzheimers-Dementia-Choosing-Residential-Care-Ts.pdf

Alzheimer's Drug Discovery Foundation. (2018). *Alzheimer's Drug Discovery Foundation*. Alzdiscovery. https://www.alzdiscovery.org/

Alzheimer's Foundation of America. (2017). *Alzheimer's Foundation of America*. Alzheimer's Foundation of America. https://alzfdn.org/

Alzheimer's Society. (2019). *Recognising when someone is reaching the end of their life*. Alzheimer's Society. https://www.alzheimers.org.uk/get-support/help-dementia-care/recognising-when-someone-reaching-end-their-life

Alzheimer's Society. (2021a, February 24). *The Progression and stages of dementia*. Alzheimer's Society. Www.alzheimers.org.uk. https://www.alzheimers.org.uk/about-dementia/symptoms-and-diagnosis/how-dementia-progresses/progression-stages-dementia

Alzheimer's Society. (2021b, September 20). *What can increase a person's risk of dementia?* Alzheimer's Society. https://www.alzheimers.org.uk/about-dementia/risk-factors-and-prevention/what-can-increase-persons-risk-of-dementia

Alzheimer's Society. (2021c, November 25). *How to reduce your risk of Alzheimer's and other dementias.* Alzheimer's Society. Www.alzheimers.org.uk. https://www.alzheimers.org.uk/about-dementia/risk-factors-and-prevention/how-reduce-your-risk-alzheimers-and-other-dementias

Alzheimer's Society. (2023b). *Feelings after a person with dementia has died.* Alzheimer's. https://www.alzheimers.org.uk/get-support/help-dementia-care/feelings-after-person-has-died

American Brain Foundation. (2019). *American Brain Foundation.* American Brain Foundation. https://www.americanbrainfoundation.org/

Amin, S. (2023, April 10). *Average monthly cost of memory care and ways to save.* Healthline. https://www.healthline.com/health/what-is-the-average-monthly-cost-for-memory-care

Better Health Channel. (n.d.-a). *Dementia - behaviour changes.* betterhealth. https://www.betterhealth.vic.gov.au/health/conditionsandtreatments/dementia-behaviour-changes#bhc-content

Better Health Channel. (2012). *Dementia - behaviour changes.* Vic.gov.au. https://www.betterhealth.vic.gov.au/health/conditionsandtreatments/dementia-behaviour-changes

Brightfocus Foundation. (2013). *Home.* BrightFocus Foundation. https://www.brightfocus.org/

Carbo, D. (2022, December 2). *Managing post traumatic caregiver stress syndrome.* Caregiver Relief. https://www.caregiverrelief.com/caregiver-stress-syndrome-symptoms/

Careforth. (2023, June 28). *The stages of Alzheimer's disease: Pre-diagnosis to late-stage dementia.* Caregiver Support and Resources. https://careforth.com/blog/the-7-stages-of-alzheimers#:~:text=Alzheimer%27s%20disease%20is%20a%20progressive%20disease%20that%20gradually%20worsens%20over

Causes Of Dementia. (2019). *Dementia.org.* Dementia.org. https://www.dementia.org/causes

CDC. (2019). *What is Alzheimer's disease?* CDC. https://www.cdc.gov/aging/index.html

Cleveland Clinic. (2022, December 30). *Acetylcholine (ACh): What it is, function*

&. deficiency. Cleveland Clinic. https://my.clevelandclinic.org/health/articles/24568-acetylcholine-ach

Compassion & Choices. (2022). *Dementia: 7 stages*. Compassion & Choices. https://www.compassionandchoices.org/resource/dementia-7-stages

Cox, J. (2022, April 29). *How long does grief last? Timelines, symptoms, and getting help*. Psych Central. https://psychcentral.com/lib/grief-healing-and-the-one-to-two-year-myth#grief-timeline

Dementia Care Collaborative. (n.d.). *MGH dementia care collaborative*. MGH Dementia Care Collaborative. Retrieved August 4, 2023, from https://dementiacarecollaborative.org/

Dementia Society of America. (2009). *Dementia society of America*. https://www.dementiasociety.org/

Dementia Society of America. (2023, July). *Definitions.*. https://www.dementiasociety.org/definitions

Dementia Spring. (2023). *Dementia spring - Helping artists tell a new story of dementia*. Dementia Spring. https://dementiaspring.org/

Dementia.org. (n.d.-a). *Symptoms of dementia*. Dementia.org. https://www.dementia.org/symptoms

Dementia.org. (n.d.-b). *Types of dementia. Better understanding your Dementia*. Dementia.org. https://www.dementia.org/types

Fletcher, A. A. (2023). *Honoring grief and coping with loss*. Psychology Today. https://www.psychologytoday.com/us/blog/keeping-it-real-and-resilient/202208/honoring-grief-and-coping-with-loss

Ford-Martin, P. (2022, August 28). *Types of Dementia*. WebMD. https://www.webmd.com/alzheimers/alzheimers-dementia#1-1

Gareth. (2021, September 23). *The seven dementia stages and how to care for them*. The CareSide. https://www.thecareside.com.au/post/the-seven-dementia-stages-and-how-to-care-for-them/#:~:text=Stage%205%3A%20Moderately%20severe%20cognitive

Hallstrom, L. (2022, October 18). *The 7 stages of dementia &. symptoms*. Www.aplaceformom.com. https://www.aplaceformom.com/caregiver-resources/articles/dementia-stages

Heather. (2015, June 10). *Caregivers suffering from PTSD (Post Traumatic Stress Disorder)*. Concierge Care Advisors. https://www.conciergecareadvisors.com/caregivers-suffering-from-ptsd/

Hospice Foundation of America. (2019). *Hospice foundation of America - Home.* Hospice Foundation of America. https://hospicefoundation.org/

John Hopkins Medicine. (2023). *The Johns Hopkins University School of Medicine.* https://www.hopkinsmedicine.org/som/

John Hopkins Medicine. (2023). *Welcome to The Johns Hopkins Hospital.* https://www.hopkinsmedicine.org/the-johns-hopkins-hospital

Johns Hopkins Medicine. (2019). *Bedsores.* Johns Hopkins Medicine. https://www.hopkinsmedicine.org/health/conditions-and-diseases/bedsores

Kelly, N. (2018, January 3). *You can't pour from an empty cup* [Tweet]. Twitter https://twitter.com/norm

LBDA. (2017). *Home | Lewy Body Dementia Association.* Lbda.org. https://www.lbda.org/

Mace, N. L., & Rabins, P. V. (2021). *The 36-Hour Day: A Family Guide to Caring for People Who Have Alzheimer's Disease and Other Dementias.* In Amazon (seventh edition). Johns Hopkins University Press.

Marley, M. (2013, August 13). *5 Things to never say to a person with Alzheimer's.* UsAgainstAlzheimer's. https://www.usagainstalzheimers.org/blog/5-things-never-say-person-alzheimers

Mayo Clinic. (2019). *Transient ischemic attack (TIA) - symptoms and causes.* Mayo Clinic. https://www.mayoclinic.org/diseases-conditions/transient-ischemic-attack/symptoms-causes/syc-20355679

Mayo Clinic. (2023). *Home.* https://www.mayoclinic.org/

Medicare.gov. (n.d.). *Home.* https://www.medicare.gov/care-compare/?redirect=true&providerType=NursingHome

Mount Sinai. (2019). *The Mount Sinai Hospital - New York City.* Mount Sinai Health System. https://www.mountsinai.org/locations/mount-sinai

National Institute on Aging. (2019). *Home.* https://www.nia.nih.gov

Neural Effects. (2023). *What can make dementia worse? (Answers to 13 FAQs).* Neural Effects. https://neuraleffects.com/blog/what-can-make-dementia-worse/

News-Medical. (2019, February 27). *Parkinson's disease history.* News-Medical.net. https://www.news-medical.net/health/Parkinsons-Disease-History.aspx

NIH. (2017). *Managing personality and behavior changes in Alzheimer's.* National Institute on Aging. https://www.nia.nih.gov/health/managing-personality-and-behavior-changes-alzheimers

Nolo. (2023). *How to settle an estate.* Www.nolo.com. https://www.nolo.com/legal-encyclopedia/how-settle-estate.html

Nuush. (2020, December 3). *"We eat first with our eyes".* Nuush. https://nuush.co.uk/we-eat-first-with-our-eyes/

Phsiopedia. (n.d.). *Global Deterioration scale.* Physiopedia. https://www.physiopedia.com/Global_Deterioration_Scale#:~:text=The%20Global%20Deterioration%20Scale%20(GDS)

Quotes For Dementia Caregivers In Need Of Inspiration | Activepro Nursing & Homecare Inc. | Niagara. (2018, July 10). *Homecare Agency | Activepro Nursing & Homecare Inc.* https://www.nursehomecare.ca/site/blog/2018/07/10/homecare-services-inspirational-quotes-for-dementia-caregivers

Robinson, L. (2018, November 2). *Home.* HelpGuide.. https://www.helpguide.org/articles/alzheimers-dementia-aging/tips-for-alzheimers-caregivers.htm

Rosalynn Carter Institute. (2020). *Rosalynn Carter Institute for Caregivers.* Https://Rosalynncarter.org/. https://rosalynncarter.org/

Sauer, A. (2019, May 6). *The 7 stages of dementia.* Retirement Resources | Leisure Care. https://www.leisurecare.com/resources/7-stages-dementia/

Schein, C. (2020, October 15). *What are the 7 stages of dementia?.* Aegis Living. https://www.aegisliving.com/resource-center/the-stages-of-caregiving-the-changes-you-will-face-with-dementia/

Schempp, D., & LCSW. (2013). *When caregiving ends.* Family Caregiver Alliance. https://www.caregiver.org/resource/when-caregiving-ends/

Snow, T. (2019). *Home.* Positive Approach to Care. https://teepasnow.com/

Social Care Institute for Excellence. (2020, March). *Carers' needs - End-of-life care and dementia.* SCIE. https://www.scie.org.uk/dementia/advanced-dementia-and-end-of-life-care/end-of-life-care/last-days-hours.asp

The DAWN Method. (n.d.). *DAWN Strength-Based Dementia Care.* The DAWN Method. https://thedawnmethod.com/

UCLA Health. (2023). *Ronald Reagan UCLA Medical Center, Los Angeles.* UCLA Health. Www.uclahealth.org. https://www.uclahealth.org/hospitals/reagan

UPMC. (n.d.). *Wandering Tendencies in Patients with Alzheimer's Disease and Dementia.* UPMC | Life Changing Medicine. https://www.upmc.com/services/seniors/resources-for-caregivers/wandering-tendencies-patients-alzheimers-dementia

WebMD. (2023). *Types of Dementia.* WebMD. https://www.webmd.com/alzheimers/alzheimers-dementia#1-1

World Health Organization. (2020, August 5). *Palliative care.* World Health Organization. https://www.who.int/news-room/fact-sheets/detail/palliative-care

World Health Organization. (2023, March 15). *Dementia.* World Health Organization. https://www.who.int/news-room/fact-sheets/detail/dementia

Printed in Great Britain
by Amazon

53595970R00095